T0269240

TELe-Health

Series editors:
Fabio Capello
Cumberland Infirmary
North Cumbria University Hospitals
Carlisle
United Kingdom

Giovanni Rinaldi
Ospedali Riuniti Marche Nord
Pesaro
Italy

Giovanna Gatti
European Institute of Oncology (IEO)
Milan
Italy

Recent advances in technology and medicine are rapidly changing the face of health care. A revolution is occurring in diagnosis and treatment thanks to the implementation of instrumentation and techniques deriving from engineering and research. In addition, a cultural conversion is taking place in which geographical and social boundaries are about to be overcome, resulting in enhanced availability and quality of care. Telemedicine has been considered a possible means of improving health care worldwide that is likely to change the way in which doctors deal with patients and diseases. While various restraints continue to limit the application of telemedicine in different settings and different areas of health, the innovations emerging from eHealth and telecare could stimulate a great leap forward for medicine, provided that some basic rules are taken into consideration and followed. In this series, diverse aspects of tele-health – preventive, promotive, and curative – will be covered by leading experts in the field with the aim of realizing the full potential of the new and exciting technological solutions at our disposal.

Giovanni Rinaldi
Editor

New Perspectives in Medical Records

Meeting the Needs of Patients and Practitioners

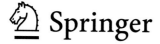 Springer

Editor
Giovanni Rinaldi
Ospedali Riuniti Marche Nord
Pesaro
Italy

ISSN 2198-6037   ISSN 2198-6045   (electronic)
TELe-Health
ISBN 978-3-319-28659-4   ISBN 978-3-319-28661-7   (eBook)
DOI 10.1007/978-3-319-28661-7

Library of Congress Control Number: 2016958442

Printed on acid-free paper

This Springer imprint is published by Springer Nature
The registered company is Springer International Publishing AG
The registered company address is: Gewerbestrasse 11, 6330 Cham, Switzerland

Preface

For a long time, governments and regional authorities have set up projects on the use of medical records for different needs: longitudinal and omni-inclusive, specialists for each medical discipline, synthetics, and for emergencies. In this context, the industry has provided its expertise and has proposed solutions to the different needs.

But, despite the enthusiastic expectations of the initiatives by governments and regional authorities, in the literature, we find criticisms, problems, and lack of understanding; the question is whether these initiatives have improved services, reduced costs, and improved care to citizens. The technology has reached a high degree of maturity, and in this context, there are users with different needs, and each of them wants to be the driver of the actions related to the production, management, processing, and use of medical records.

So, whereas policy makers (with the reason on their side) believe that technology can make improvements and they produce rules and regulations that in some cases are accompanied by incentives, the industry, however, continues to produce solutions to solve temporary needs, always looking for new initiatives imposed by politicians or health managers. Doctors (they are the main users of these systems – not to be forgotten) have gained skills and needs that must be taken into account. If you did not, from their point of view, the creation of clinical tools and applications is not in line with the care needs.

In this context, for some years, patients enter the medical record world, and they correctly pretend that their needs must be taken into consideration. They are not only users but also the protagonists of the process of care. In the technological workflow, patients want a role in the management of clinical information – they claim as their own – and as part of privacy context. They want access to information and, in some cases, to complete clinical and social data, they search for "collaboration" with other patients through social applications, and they need interaction with the doctors and health staff.

And finally, we must not forget the many initiatives proposed by the European Commission, in terms of investments in innovation and improvement of technologies in the health sector. These projects have improved communication between researchers, the technology, and the needs of those who use these tools.

It is hard not to take into account all the needs expressed by the various components involved in this complex, articulated ecosystem. But it seems that it is not enough. The result, according to the literature, remains the same: close to some clear successes, in some cases, there is disaffection and disinterest and in other cases frustrations and tensions. According to some authors, national programs have not always kept their promises; they do not always document cost reduction and the improvements of clinical results are not always well proved from surveys. When cases of success are documented, they are often accompanied by delays, higher costs, and lower results.

Web 2.0 has brought innovative concepts in the ICT landscape, and also in the health context, we note the entrance of solutions driven by these concepts: sharing, collaboration, open source, pervasive computing, user engagement, distribute knowledge, pervasive and participative actions, and networks of communities.

But around users' needs and to the novelty brought by technology, new clinical models are appearing, such as precision medicine, system medicine, cross-border care, access to international centers of clinical excellence, networks of pathology, and care of chronic disease, and we wonder how can traditional medical records face the complexity of this rich ecosystem?

Perhaps we need to rethink what has been done, not forgetting the good practices and the countless progress. We have to consider that many medical records are affected by an old design although there have been many advances. These advances should be combined with the proposed innovations: creating medical records starting with the doctor-patient relationship, improving the understanding and usability of clinical information provided to patients, and enhancing and promoting infrastructures as really federative in which collaboration between the actors is the norm.

Medical records are complex living objects. They require new impulses according to the new demands made by the actors of the eHealth ecosystem.

Traditional medical records do not meet the new requirements expressed by new clinical models and by the advent of new technologies. The result is amply demonstrated and discussed in many articles published in specialized magazines.

We want this collection of contributions to be the first step toward a new way of thinking about the design and development of medical records: it is a provocation for further discussions.

The book is an opportunity for the reflection, the discussion, and the understanding that can inspire new attitudes, modify directions, improve the vision, and propose ideas for a concrete and fruitful work.

Next to traditional solutions, we will also explore new concepts and new models that are more responsive to the changing needs of the actors of the health system.

And it is these traditional experiences that have worked so well until now that due to the advent of these new features, they require themselves to change direction. We argue that medical records must be designed from the doctor-patient relationship and that the concepts of sharing, collaboration, and pervasive knowledge should be taken into account.

Moreover, the needs of the patients must be taken into account also; the patient empowerment concept must be supported by suitable tools (unfortunately still missing), tools that can present clinical data to patients in a way that they can understand them.

New medical models like precision medicine and system medicine need to treat a large amount of data; therefore mathematical algorithms must be used in order to extract knowledge from data.

At last, in the complex clinical pathways that the new medical models require, a set of different agencies and medical institutions are engaged in working together, so medical records must respond to the requirements expressed by a multiagency environment.

These reasons impose the choice of new infrastructure and push toward models of federative architecture.

Pesaro, Italy   Giovanni Rinaldi

Introduction. Medical Records: Are We at the Top? Is There Still Room for Innovation?

In literature, there are a lot of publications about medical records or health IT [1, 2]. On the one hand, we note the presentation of standard applications and architectures, also very often accompanied by evidence of few successes especially as it regards the major national projects, but on the other side, we note that there are emerging new ideas and new concepts that are being born and are taking new roads.

What I would say is that there is a world still very overwhelmed that communicates not always and not just through academic journals but through "informal" communication, blogs, tweets, and so on. I think it is more correct to call the area they are treating as Health 2.0 or eHealth [3].

In the last years, it seems we are attending at a new era of health IT. In it, we note great emphasis in innovation and new paradigms are tested and proposed. Often this novelty is drawn by the world called Web 2.0 [4] (transported in the health world, the correct term is Health 2.0) in which the concepts of sharing, open source, collaboration, user engagement, pervasive computing, distribute knowledge, pervasive and participative actions, and network of communities are enhanced.

Obviously also new devices and hardware have contributed to this further ICT revolution especially as regards the opportunity offered by mobile devices and telemedicine instruments: with those devices and applications, "everyone" can claim or monitor health status, manage clinical workflow, and treat medical data.

Whereas before it was about checking and analyzing the processes (through software and hardware) according to the standard medical applications proposed by the software industry, now the paradigm seems changed: emphasis is posed on the users such as what counts, what is useful, and what is needed, and all of that are through new technologies that allow the passage of the focus from the processes to the users.

User needs and user expectations produce relationships, and these are mediated and in some cases enhanced by the technology; for this reason, it is much more than a "system," and we are speaking about a health information space: an "ecosystem."

In this ecosystem, medical data are driven by the mechanism of publication–brokerage–delivery: publication consists in the actions for which the doctor managing the clinical data of a patient allows access to other clinicians who need to access them for care reasons; brokerage allows to drive the information according to the care right for the patient, and it has a meaning of setting the rules of technical functions in the usage of clinical data; delivery consists in the need to access information according to different meanings (medical care, social care, health education, etc.) driven by different needs according to the patient, the doctors, the health researcher, and the policy maker.

But all of this makes sense if it is governed: privacy must assure the patients and not stop or complicate the care; the concept of data property in health assumes a different concept compared to the management of money in Internet banking procedures or journey booking and entertainment online.

In the ecosystem, information (as actor relationship) has value and is transacted in the delivery of care, so the development of services and the deployment of clinical capabilities and practice through the conversational relationships among the actors produce and enrich the medical information value chain, but inevitably, they are recognized as a cooperation of a set of roles that came with their own responsibilities, performing publication, brokerage, and delivery of clinical information.

We inscribe the complex relationships among the actors in an environment supporting the operation and governance of a dynamic and participative ecosystem of care, in which many actors, belonging to different institutions, agencies, and organizations, depend on each other and interact and transact in complex ways over the infrastructure and in the real, face-to-face world where resources and policies emerge and evolve, but because there are hard limits on capacities and resources, optimization and rationing are realities that must be faced, while costs and demand are managed.

Clinical information is constructed upon relationships between the actors. The value-adding chain, on which health transactions are based in health information economy, is founded on these acts of communication, and it collects a set of roles and interactions working together to create and deliver a service, in which each element provides its own contribution for the benefit of the users adding "value" inside the ecosystem.

So the construction of information according to the roles and its interpretation assumes a fundamental role in the design of the medical record.

Clinical information produced in this ecosystem fosters collaboration among users and can be intentional or accidental, because it is based on the meaning of the information created: social collaboration among health actors is based on voluntary traditional clinical information sharing, but there is a great amount of medical information produced for some scopes that can be reused, revealing hidden connection among data. This promotes accidental collaboration, unthinkable in the past.

But the ecosystem described, wherein the relationships among the actors belonging to different organizations, institutions, and agencies live and are nurtured (even if they want to continue to express their ethos in the collaborative work that a medical job requires), gives rise to new technology architectures and promotes the realization of federative platforms, in which clinical information and services are shared, fostering also collaboration and the inclusion in the care workflow of all the actors including the "empowered" patient.

So the first concept of this innovation is a new look at how the clinical data is composed, starting from the relationship among the actors and based on the set of rules depending on the different agencies where the actors belong. In a clear manner, the role of the actors assumes an important function in the ecosystem and needs to be governed. Let us take a look at the process of care describing the access to a medical excellence center as study case [5]. The patient accessing the medical excellence center brings with him all the referrals, reports, results, and medical notes made in different medical centers obviously in different electronic formats. During access in the center, clinicians will record clinical data (in different formats we presume), and when the patient is discharged, the follow-up done by the local health organization must maintain the contact with the specialized doctors in the excellence center. The main intuition is to exchange data in different formats, but very often, the software procedures are not standard and, even if these are declared as standard, in reality they are "dialects" of the standard.

The process of data exchanging is more complicated if the medical excellence center is abroad.

In this workflow, organizational processes done in different organizations that inevitably must meet the patients are well defined, but what about the information? What about the needs of the patients, doctors, and researchers? What about the empowerment of the patient? Can the patient communicate easily with all the doctors involved in the care? While it is considering the valid organizational and economic considerations, we agree that something is missing.

Let us think also of the network of pathologies or the management of chronic disease: the processes are different to that described, but the need of sharing clinical data is the same.

While the clinical processes listed now are made of relations that produce information and require the sharing of information, the creation of a network, and real patient engagement, we wonder how is it possible with the current tools?

These concepts introduce the idea of the actors. There is no relationship without the actors. Whereas, as said, the traditional medical records are based on the processes in the health system and finalized within the walls of the organization, strong emphasis must be posed on the actors: clinicians (including nurses and other medical operators), patients and their families, researchers, and policy makers. Each of them is part of the ecosystem, each of them produces information that must be shared for the benefit of all, and each of them has their own needs and requirements.

Could the focus on the clinical data based on relationships and the attention to the clinical narrative be enough?

What can the actors (doctors, patients, researchers, policy makers) do about this amount of data?

We are subject to a kind of "pollution caused by data." But it is better to get information rather than not have them. The point is how can we use them profitably?

There is in literature a great emphasis on big data and also in medicine. But what is most remarkable is that very often, in medicine, paradigms of use of big data typical of other areas are assumed.

In the ecosystem described, a lot of clinical and medical-social data are produced. Moreover the new paradigms brought by Health 2.0 foster the production of information by all the actors. Mobile devices, the instrument for communication in telemedicine (the m-Health area), produce information that must be analyzed; the empowerment of the patient produces information; the accessing of all the actors to specific social networks produces information; the new medical instruments used for monitoring or providing diagnosis produce information; the recent advances in genomics and the connection with the diagnosis formulation or care processes produce information.

So that this amount of "different" types of information could be fruitful, it is not enough to be shared in the ecosystem (as we described so far), but it must be provided suitable algorithms and methodologies to make the information useful.

We are not just thinking about the usage of algorithms but also, for example, the presentation of the data to the actors.

It is common practice in health to exchange data as they are generated. So referrals are presented to patients in the form that they are analyzed by doctors. In many situations, it can be difficult for patients to catch what counts for them.

By the way this is another mismatching about the property of data; certainly the medical document or the referral is the property of the patient but what can be the aim if it is not understood?

We are not asserting that it is not convenient to show the referrals to the patient but just to present them in a way that is understandable. Fortunately researchers [6, 7] and institutions are studying opportunities and instruments to make the clinical data comprehensible to patients. It is the case of the challenge supported by Health Design Challenge [8, 9].

In the site, almost 40 projects in which clinical data are presented to the patient in a comprehensible way are shown. The results are very remarkable.

The TedMed conference by Thomas Goetz by the title "It Is Time to Redesign Medical Data" is another example in which the concept of promoting broadens patient participation through a clear and understandable vision of the patient's own clinical data with the aim of arranging well-organized medical strategies and enhancing suitable health education [10].

He affirms that "Your medical chart: it's hard to access, impossible to read – and full of information that could make you healthier if you just knew how to use it."

This is the point of view of the patient; I think it is essential for patient empowerment.

But what about the point of view of the researcher or the clinician?

In recent years, precision medicine and system medicine have been proposed as new medical models. Precision medicine is an emerging approach for disease treatment and prevention that takes into account individual variability in genes, environment, and lifestyle for each person [11].

These approaches are based on the systems perspective in order to consider the holistic and composite characteristics of a clinical problem and evaluate the problem with the use of computational and mathematical tools [12, 13].

For this reason, a coordinated approach across disciplines and across research and industry and among all the relevant stakeholders is required. The underlying concept regards the creation of a network in which system biology, practice information, and environmental information are shared in a broader system biology and clinical community.

Those medical models are based on the idea that the treatments are driven by data and each patient is unique so treatment must be personalized [14].

In these models, the concepts already treated previously about the collaboration between doctors and researchers through the creation of networks, a new vision about the usage and inclusion of genetic data and the integration with clinical data and environmental data, and a new look to the relationship between patients and doctors by considering also narrative medicine as intentional information are enhanced; in addition, as we said previously, this information reveals hidden correlations among data, and this promotes accidental collaboration previously unimaginable to study. Then at last it becomes necessary to the implementation of suitable algorithms for analyzing and extracting useful information by the great amount of data.

We wonder: could precision medicine be fruitful, nurtured, and enhanced using the current medical record?

Big data in medicine therefore is not just management of a great amount of data but also algorithms and methodologies of analysis.

In conclusion, these concepts are the base of the ecosystem we are describing: the relationship between the actors of the ecosystem; the role of each of them also belonging to different agencies; the creation of networks between the actors; the social interactions; the medical doctor relationship and the approach to the narrative medicine; the need of personalized care; the integration between genetic data, practice data, and environmental data; the need to make information accessible and comprehensible; the complexity of the voluntary and accidental collaboration; and the usage of complex algorithms in order to analyze data.

They are supported by the concepts of sharing, collaboration, publication, brokerage, delivery, and governance.

And so that these needs can be accepted, it is necessary to have a new vision about medical data in order to face the challenge that modern healthcare requires: system medicine, precision medicine, pathology networks, chronic disease care, the access to medical excellence centers, and cross-border care.

Pesaro, Italy   Giovanni Rinaldi

References

1. Greenhalgh T, Potts HW, Wong G, Bark P, Swinglehurst D (2009) Tensions and paradoxes in electronic patient record research: a systematic literature review using the meta-narrative method. Milbank Q 87(4):729–788. doi:10.1111/j.1468-0009.2009.00578.x
2. Hayrinen K, Saranto K, Nykanen P (2008) Definition, structure, content, use and impacts of electronic health records: a review of the research literature. Int J Med Inform 77:291–304
3. Van De Belt TH, Engelen LJ, Berben SAA, Schoonhoven L (2010) Definition of Health 2.0 and Medicine 2.0: a systematic review. J Med Internet Res 12(2):e18
4. O'Reilly T. What is Web 2.0? O'Reilly Media. [Online] Available from http://oreilly.com/web2/archive/what-is-web-20.html. Accessed 9 Oct 2015

5. Rinaldi G (2014) An introduction to the technological basis of eHealth. In: Gaddi A et al (eds) eHealth, care and quality of life. Springer, Italia, pp 31–67. doi:10.1007/978-88-470-5253-6_3

6. Blake Lesselroth J, Pieczkiewicz DS (2012) Data visualization strategies for the electronic health record. In: Berhardt Leon V (ed) Advances in medicine and biology, vol 16. Nova Science Publishers, Inc. Hauppauge NY USA

7. VAHC (2013) Proceedings of the 2013 workshop on visual analytics in healthcare. Washington, DC. www.visualanalyticshealthcare.org

8. http://healthdesign.devpost.com/

9. http://healthdesignchallenge.com/

10. http://www.ted.com/talks/thomas_goetz_it_s_time_to_redesign_medical_data

11. National Academy of Science (2011) Toward precision medicine: building a knowledge network for biomedical research and a new taxonomy of disease. The National Academies Press, Washington, DC

12. Ahn AC, Tewari M, Poon CS, Phillips RS (2006) The limits of reductionism in medicine: could systems biology offer an alternative? PLoS Med 3(6):e208. doi:10.1371/journal. pmed.0030208

13. Ahn AC, Tewari M, Poon CS, Phillips RS (2006) The clinical applications of a systems approach. PLoS Med 3(7):e209. doi:10.1371/journal. pmed.0030209

14. Collins FS, Varmus H (2015) A new initiative on precision medicine. N Engl J Med 372:793–795. doi:10.1056/NEJMp1500523

Contents

EHR, EPR, PS, PHR: Different Medical Records for Different Aims: Roles of Doctors, Patients, and Institutions

Giovanni Rinaldi

1.1 Introduction

It seems we are approaching a new information and communications technology (ICT) era in the health context: we note that new ideas are emerging and new concepts are being born. These innovations come in two types, strictly linked together: hardware and software.

The web2.0 has brought about innovative concepts in the ICT framework, and also in the health context we note the arrival of solutions driven by these concepts, such as sharing, collaboration, open source, pervasive computing, user engagement, distributed knowledge, pervasive and participative actions, and networks of communities.

Obviously, the introduction of new devices has also contributed to this revolution, especially in regard to the opportunities offered by mobile devices and telemedicine instruments. With these devices everyone can claim access to clinical data and require access to clinical pathways, then being able to send to professionals the data sourced from telemedicine instruments for monitoring their own health status [1].

In a recent post Eric Topol declares http://www.huffingtonpost.com/eric-j-topol-md/health-technology_b_1610684.html "Take your electrocardiogram on your smartphone and send it to your doctor. Have a suspicious skin lesion that might be cancer? Just take a picture with your smartphone and you can have a quick test back in minutes. Does your child have an ear infection? Just get the scope attachment to your smartphone and get a 10× magnified high-resolution view of your child's ear-drums and send them for automatic detection of whether antibiotics will be needed. Worried about glaucoma? You can get a contact lens with an embedded chip that continuously measures eye pressure and transmits data to your phone. These are just

G. Rinaldi
Ospedali Riuniti Marche Nord, Pesaro, Italy
e-mail: rinaldi8giovanni@gmail.com

© Springer International Publishing Switzerland 2017
G. Rinaldi (ed.), *New Perspectives in Medical Records*, TELe-Health,
DOI 10.1007/978-3-319-28661-7_1

a few examples of the innovative smartphone software and hardware that have been developed and will soon be available for broad use." Moreover, in the book "The patient will see you now" [2] Topol affirms that we are moving in a new direction towards a world in which each individual will have all their own medical data and the computer power to process it in the context of their own world, and there will be comprehensive medical information about a person that is easily accessible, analyzable, and transferable. People engaged in the medical process (both professionals and patients) can produce much clinical data, and can access information on worldwide networks.

In the digitally connected world, smart devices and applications are ubiquitous, and we wonder whether this pervasive digitalization will lead to better healthcare for people.

These advances encourage new approaches to clinical practice, medical research, and medicine; generally speaking, they prompt professional collaboration and patient engagement, but they also raise questions and pose challenges for existing healthcare delivery systems.

On the other hand, we are also witnessing the introduction of new clinical models. Two such models are precision medicine and system medicine.

Precision medicine "refers to the tailoring of medical treatment to the individual characteristics of each patient. It does not literally mean the creation of drugs or medical devices that are unique to a patient, but rather the ability to classify individuals into subpopulations that differ in their susceptibility to a particular disease or their response to a specific treatment. Preventive or therapeutic interventions can then be concentrated on those who will benefit, sparing expense and side effects for those who will not" [3].

System medicine is prospective medicine that will be predictive, personalized, preventive, and participatory [4], and that will take into account the multiple components of the healthcare system, including disease outcomes as reported by the patients themselves, and as reported by public and private organizations involved in healthcare management [5]. System medicine is beginning to explore medicine beyond linear relationships and single parameters, and involves multiple parameters obtained across multiple time points and spatial conditions to achieve a holistic perspective of an individual [6].

System medicine provides the best available care for each individual, and it also requires that researchers and healthcare providers have access to large sets of health- and disease-related data linked to individual patients [7].

In the same way, precision medicine is designed to provide the best accessible care for each individual; however, this is not achievable without a massive reorientation of the information systems on which researchers and healthcare providers depend: these systems, like the medicine they wish to support, must be individualized.

So precision medicine is an emerging approach for disease treatment and prevention that takes into account individual variability in genes, environment, and lifestyle for each person.

These medical models are based on the idea that the treatments are driven by data, and as each patient is unique so the treatment must be personalized.

These medical models tend to overcome the traditional reductionism in medicine (in which treatments are focused on components where information about time, space, and context can be lost) in favor of a system of medicine where emphasis is placed on the interrelationships between dynamic and individualized multidimensional medical treatments.

The necessity for treating huge amounts of information (molecular information, lifestyle, environment, clinical data) with adequate mathematical instruments and algorithms emerges clearly from these new medical models.

Research in the medical context in the past decade has made important steps in the identification of better methods for the care of patients, and has produced strong specialization to cope with different pathologies.

From a medical-organizational point of view, this specialization has brought about the realization of medical centers of excellence. These centers are especially focused on clinical specialties and inevitably have become centers of attraction for patients from different locations (also from abroad); so they are also centers of attraction for the best doctors and for the most innovative medical technologies. To access medical centers of excellence, patients must make many specific visits and undergo a number of diagnostic investigations to verify their possible access to the center. Often during this workflow the patient feels alone, and at discharge time the return home is fraught with anxieties, fears, and questions, and the follow-up risks may not be clearly explained. The context of the provision of these highly specialized clinical services is, by nature, very dynamic and requires the partnership of various bodies—including mixed public-private-voluntary organizations—which should be based on collaborative work among stakeholders from different agencies and different levels of specialization.

The context of cross-border care presents the same challenges; although the European Commission [8] wants to promote cooperation between member states on healthcare matters and has proposed directives to guarantee the safety, quality, and efficiency of care that a patient will receive in another European Union member state, the principles concerning cooperation between the organizations responsible for medical records in cross-border care seem dated and inadequate. And so it seems that the European networks of disease control and the European networks for the treatment of chronic diseases suffer from the inadequacies of the current technical systems and their inability to exchange clinical information.

In these medical models clinical information is fragmented in different organizations; each of them collects the information needed for the execution of their part of the workflow and only in some cases are clinical data exchanged through actions allowing the duplication of information.

The organizational workflows depicted above are characterized by strong collaboration between the professionals belonging to different health organizations, hospitals, and patient agencies (also including social workers, patients, and their families); they have distinct organizational aims and different infrastructures, and very often clinical data are locked in silos. In this landscape, despite the request for "working together", the dispersive vision of care predominates, tied to territorial assistance. It seems more appropriate that a clinical network organization should be really patient-centric and focused on a medical community of stakeholders belonging to different hospital or health organizations, based on the sharing of clinical information and online services.

Beyond the good intentions, the entire system does not seem prepared to address these challenges from a technical point of view; thus, instead of the innovations and the new technology era increasing collaboration, it seems that these factors increase confusion.

What is emerging in the encounter between the new technologies—in which the concepts of collaboration between the actors and the pervasive knowledge are enhanced —and the new medical models—in which communities of actors are created who share information and who will utilize huge amounts of structured and unstructured data—is the complexity of clinical information. Clinical information is a thriving entity created, managed, and nurtured by a community of users with a set of needs emerging from their access to it. We cannot allow clinical information to exist as a structured database with low-level communication tools.

It is here that we need to introduce the notion of a health ecosystem. This ecosystem is based on clear concepts, such as the plurality of actors and their relationships, and specifically the doctor-patient relationship, produces value. The utility of data in such an ecosystem depends on the users' ability and capacity to interpret it and propose conclusions; therefore, before taking any actions, it is necessary to know the value of the ecosystem: the clinical information.

1.2   The eHealth Ecosystem and Its Intrinsic Value

The complex ecosystem we have partially described consists of a set of actors belonging to different agencies governed by different aims and with their own culture and ethos.

The ecosystem comprises a set of roles and interactions working together to create and deliver services, in which each element provides its own contribution for the benefit of the users, adding "value" inside the ecosystem.

User needs and user expectations produce relationships and these are mediated and in some cases enhanced by the technology; for this reason, more than "system" we are speaking about a health information space: an "ecosystem".

The ecosystem is founded on the voluntary acts of relationship generating information; the transactions of the ecosystem are the relationships between the actors, and mainly the doctor-patient relationship.

The value of this ecosystem is the information.

The ecosystem exists and is nurtured in the information space, in which the clinical information value chain consists of voluntary acts of "publication, brokerage, and delivery". These acts, on which clinical information is based, are necessary for making available medical records and for creating a virtual community of actors, creating effective and real collaboration among the individuals interested in the healthcare context, including the patient.

We refer to "publication" because the longitudinal, holistic, comprehensive clinical information referring to a patient consists of various acts of relationship between doctor and patient and also between doctors and doctors on behalf of the patient; the outcomes of these acts must be available.

We refer to "brokerage" intending the term to mean the mechanism of making available the needed information, for the care aim, to different actors who need to use it inside the ecosystem, with ethical intent.

We refer to "delivery" in the context of establishing a network of service supply relationships of many different sorts with significant elements of trust and dependence [9].

Information consists of a set of "pieces" obtained from relationships, ordered according to the meaning of the connection between the actors.

These transactions form the relationships among the actors, and produce value and enrich the whole information ecosystem, in which actors, institutions, agencies, and organizations share medical information, build collaborations, and create virtual communities. And we should not forget that these opportunities and challenges, unthinkable some years ago, are now made possible by the new developments in technology. These developments allow pervasive computing, shared information, and distributed knowledge; collaborative tools that make available sophisticated and complex algorithms for information analysis. All of this, across agencies, institutions, and nations, empowers the creation of communities of actors engaged in the treatment of clinical information for the individual.

But at the same time, we are also aware that certain uses of technology can lead to a drift, making possible the use of incorrect forms of "do-it-yourself healthcare". For this reason, technology must be governed in the healthcare context, and this assertion is not contrary to the new development of technology.

This issue of governance is related to the concept of what are the basic clinical data units, or, in other words, the extent to which the narrative of the record can be safely broken down into such units. This seems to contrast with the database concept of real facts translated into entities, and their attributes, in the traditional data model. Moreover, all clinical observations that are recorded are situated in the context of some health problems that are being treated through the sequence of clinical encounters, conversations, relationships, and explanations of data obtained from clinical services.

This view is based on the practice of primary care, where the doctor-patient conversation, and the generated narrative, are central. This picture is somewhat different in a hospital-based acute care encounter, where the execution of medical services and the generation of clinical data are common. Here, at the clinical level, the assumption is that this relationship is episodic; it has a beginning (the hospital admission) and it will end in the patient's discharge.

So, at last, clinical information produced in the ecosystem fosters collaboration among users. This can be intentional or accidental, because it is based on the meaning of the information created: social collaboration among health actors is based on the voluntary sharing of traditional clinical information, but a great amount of medical information produced for some purposes can be reused. In addition, this information reveals connections among data, and this promotes accidental collaboration that was previously unthinkable.

The relationship between the actors produces information that is constituted by sign and meaning. A sign is always connected to a meaning. All human beings use a mechanism to make sense of the world; by means of this they give a sense to things, and when something has a meaning, that something becomes a sign for us. Sign and meaning, therefore, are strictly connected and must be considered as combined [10].

But semiotics is not just the study of signs; it is the study of signs and meanings joined together. Thus, a system of signs (a semiotic system) is always made up of at least two distinct bodies: a system of entities that we call signs and a body of features that represent their meanings.

The conversation between the actors in the ecosystem produces signs and their meanings, but the link between sign and meaning, consecutively, creates a new entity, which is their relationship.

A sign has some degree of independence and stands for something that is other than itself, i.e., there is no deterministic relationship between sign and meaning. If we consider human languages we find that often they give different names to the same object, precisely because there is no necessary connection between names and objects.

Therefore, in the ecosystem we are describing, the connection between signs and meanings is not necessarily linked. The connection can be established only by conventional rules; the rules of a code. Two independent entities—signs and meanings—are connected by the conventional rules of a code.

There is always an agent that produces signs, meanings, and conventions; we are introducing the concept of coding; in other words, the rules of the code are defined by the actors involved.

The clinical conversation is relatively simple. Two or more actors enter a relationship and exchange signs, which have meanings through the conventional rules of a code. We can document sets of relationships. The doctor-patient relationship is the main one, but in the ecosystem, the clinical information is a result of the relationships of other actors. The doctor-doctor relationship is another possibility on behalf of a patient. Three other possibilities are patient-researcher and doctor-researcher relationships in a medical research context, and policy maker-doctor in the context of an organization and the managing of resources. And, finally there is the patient-patient relationship. Obviously many other stakeholder relationships are possible, but they are not mentioned here.

Each of these relationships has the power to produce information in the ecosystem, and each of them has rules and is developed in a different way; each relationship has clear features, and for each of them we can have different signs, meanings, and codes. But all contribute to a unique purpose: patient care.

When two actors in the ecosystem enter a relationship they exchange (in reality) data (with meaning) and concepts, expressed in a narrative way or in a dialogue.

During a relationship between doctor and patient, the doctor exchanges data and concepts: signs and meanings joined by a code, whereas the patient exchanges concepts in a narrative way or in a dialogue, with these concepts inevitably having a different basis from those of the doctor. The doctor translates through their own code, eliminating possible redundancies.

This exchange differs in different cultures and depends on the ethos of the actors, with the patient-patient relationship being governed by a different code from that used in the doctor-doctor relationship. In these relationships, as predicted by the mathematician C.E. Shannon in his theory of information [11], we have to consider the entropy generated as the upper limit of the information treated, and we are also faced with a kind of noise. But we are invited to overcome the noise and maintain entropy within acceptable limits in order to recover the original information.

In the eHealth ecosystem, information is generated and interpreted in the context of determined conversations in relationships of care. By this we mean actors with roles, responsibilities, and relationships interacting and transacting in order to perform those roles and discharge those responsibilities.

The result is a complex web of conversations that take place over space and time and generate units of information that can have different meanings and significances in the different contexts and in different relationships between the actors. The conversation not only has different purposes but different sorts of purposes, such as care, management, collaboration, charity, governance, and research.

If the conversation is constrained in a set of data governed by traditional data schema, there is the risk of a loss of the meaning of the relationship. However, the power of the narrative introduces important considerations: the relationship is a voluntary act that generates information that is immediately usable, and it is collaborative, but in the narrative involuntary knowledge is hidden and it can be used in the future for other opportunities for the patient's care.

This is the limit observed in the traditional frameworks, in that so-called middleware tools can exchange data, but not clinical information.

We know that there is a necessity to group data extracted by information, but we know that this action is subject to the noise and entropy described by Shannon; this action responds to a reductionist concept of medicine, but it really works immediately.

But we should not preclude the opportunity to go to the bottom, as suggested by Richard Feynman: "There is plenty of room at the bottom" he asserted, and even if this suggestion was originally made in relation to the immense possibilities offered by miniaturization, this idea of Feynman's is should also be taken into account in the theory of information [12].

These concerns lead us to consider the narrative as the unit of information in the ecosystem more appropriate than the traditional approach and to open new opportunities.

The relationships between the actors produce intentional collaboration and intentional information. However, informational collaboration is accidental: it is obtained when clinical information created for one purpose is found and used, or when such information influences another purpose (within the limits imposed by ethics and inherent to patient care). We have introduced the concept of the act of publication to render this repurposing of clinical information as ethical under the principles of consent. This commits us to the building of an environment where the re-use of information for medical research and practice is consistently enabled and where collaboration among the stakeholders—across time, experience, and context—becomes the norm.

In the theory of clinical conversation we have pointed out that when new medical models are practiced, different medical professionals come into play in the care of the patient, and very often they belong to different organizations. In this space different relationships are introduced that create a set of conversations that produce clinical information.

1.3   The Actors and Their Needs

In the traditional design and implementation of software instruments in the health context, including medical records, the focus is placed on the organization of the services. In order to manage resources, what counts is the description and management of each step of the organizational workflow. This is the aim of enterprise resource planning (ERP), born in the commercial or industrial context; the healthcare area also has taken inspiration from these models. Obviously, during the medical workflow clinical data are stored, retrieved, and managed.

Special applications, such as patient management, patient logistics, hospital finance, and general management of the organization, have been developed and integrated so that the ERP system fits with the hospital situation and requests.

This software facilitates the integration of all the functional information flows across the organization into a single package with a common database, including the clinical data collected during patient care and now also accessible by a patient menu.

Therefore, ERP in the clinical context or in medical record applications manages the information referring to the health state of the patient according the concept of patient-centered design, in which the data are structured according to the patient's needs.

So, inside the same health organization, or in a network of health centers, or inside a region in which hospitals use the same software system (e.g., ERP, medical records) the patient data could be managed in a centralized way (or exchanged without problems), achieving what is often claimed as the desired purpose: a patient-centered system.

According to the definition provided by the Institute of Medicine (IOM), patient-centered care concerns "Providing care that is respectful of and responsive to individual patient preferences, needs, and values, and ensuring that patient values guide all clinical decisions" [13].

We want to emphasize that the meaning that technicians offer for the term "patient-centered" is regarded as not far from the meaning assumed by clinicians.

But the reality is different and this problem is just amplified by the new technologies.

The medical models described system medicine, precision medicine, enhance the concept of collaboration, which is not reflected in the use of technology.

Each relevant software application claims to be "patient-centric"; the data structure allows the assignment of data and services to the patients; if a whole system could be built for managing all the resources available, the clinical information referring to the patients, which is retrieved, compiled, and managed during the course of the clinical pathway, would be assigned to the patient and not to the management functions.

The software industry produces really unified systems with seamless modules that use a single database to store and share all patient records; these technologies also provide interoperable features with legacy and future applications; all features are available within the same organizations or the same regions adopting the same system.

The solutions enable physicians, nurses, and other authorized users to share data and streamline processes across an entire organization. An online "digital chart" displays up-to-date patient information in real time, complete with decision-support tools for physicians and nurses. Simple prompts allow swift and accurate ordering, documentation, and billing (for examples see [14, 15]).

Although these are excellent tools from the traditional point of view, we think that we can do something more.

When we analyze the new medical models described before, we can identify a paradox.

Each software application is patient-centered. In the complex workflows described previously, in which different medical centers or hospitals are engaged in the new medical models, each of them is really patient-centered within the same organization. The paradox is that we have a number of centers instead of one, depending on the organization that is engaged in curing the patient. The patient is considered the center within each organization, but he or she has the need to be considered the center of their own pathology. When the cure is fragmented in different organizations problems arise because of the centrality of clinical information.

With this patient-centric concept, there are strong motivations towards the introduction of the eHealth architecture that we will analyze below.

The distinction we are introducing here is between infrastructural approaches following the needs of the actors and applications-oriented approaches; the distinction is not always so clear cut in reality.

All business systems or health information systems are mixed. They provide different levels and intensities of process orientation and needs for actors' orientation. They, and the platforms that deliver them, also join structural and infrastructural elements: both application and service-oriented components. But we emphasize that the process orientation often does not take into account the centrality of the patient in the course of different episodes of care, both isolated and integrated with each other, and it also omits the needs of the actors.

But what we want to highlight now is that, beyond the good intentions, the vaunted centrality of the patient is not supported by technology.

This circumstance raises the issues of the meaning that each actor in the eHealth ecosystem provides for every action.

Each actor in the ecosystem has needs and requirements that must be taken into account. This is what new technologies are emphasizing.

The introduction of new concepts such as sharing, collaboration, open source, pervasive computing, user engagement, distributed knowledge, pervasive and participative actions, and networks of communities; the advent of mobile health (mHealth) solutions; and the emerging of new clinical models based on professional collaboration, sharing knowledge, and persistent information, invite us to move the focus of the problem from the organizational motivations towards the needs of the users.

We are seeing a shift in the heart of the problem of the design, development, and implementation of eHealth solutions, from the clinical organizational workflow to what counts for the actors in the ecosystem; i.e., what is useful and what is needed.

This different point of view introduces the concepts of actors and their needs: who are the subjects interested in and involved in the production, the use, the delivery, and the management of clinical information?

In the ecosystem we note a plurality of actors. They are characterized by clear features depending on their behaviors and depending on their belonging to an agency with organizational rules.

As described, the modern clinical models foster collaborations between stakeholders belonging to different health organizations. These collaborations generate clinical information (as we have already seen) referring to a patient.

The main need of the professionals involved in the care of the patient is collaboration. This feature is not a necessity for complex models. During the workflow describing the access to a medical center of excellence, different doctors contribute to the care of the patient, and this is so also for the network of pathologies or for the care of chronic diseases. But this concept is also valid for general practice. General practitioners (GPs) are the centers of collaboration networks that involve specialists. If we take a look at medical research, the landscape is not different. Collaboration is the main activity that involves, in some cases, specialists, GPs, and also patients.

In all these models, GPs, nurses, specialists, social workers, patients, families of the patients, and researchers are involved in a collaboration network. Each of them has their own responsibilities, needs, and hopes, and they belong to different organizational units.

Each actor contributes to the value of the ecosystem, producing clinical information. This information is based on voluntary acts of relationships between the actors. Each relationship involves different actors: each one has different signs, meanings, and rules and different codes. Each relationship is characterized by data, their interpretation and explanation, and narrative.

Now we can have a brief look at some needs expressed by some actors in the system.

1.3.1   The Needs of the Patients and Their Families

In the past decade, mostly pushed by technology, patients have reached high levels of awareness about their own health state, including factors such as lifestyle, health education, and knowledge of their own pathologies.

Different cultural movements have arisen with the aim of explaining the basis of this engagement. Most of them point out the free initiative of the patient against the power of traditional medicine. The process has been explained as a type of dis-mediation (apomediation) [16], in which the patient searches for information on the network, tending to replace the doctor, or to integrate (from their point of view) the information released by the doctor.

Moreover, patients are encouraged to take an active part in their own health management.

The engagement of the patient in the care process is considered as a new meth-odology of healthcare that proceeds from the perspective that optimal outcomes of healthcare interventions are achieved when patients become active participants in the healthcare process. The center of this philosophy is the importance of individual involvement in health decision-making [17].

So we now come to Telecare—the application of information and communication technologies in health and care, encompassing curative, preventive, and promotional aspects, as well as the interaction between doctor and patient—allowing patients to monitor their own health state. Moreover, telemonitoring devices are making it easier for healthcare providers to evaluate the health status of patients without an office visit, and data-monitoring centers can alert the clinician to significant changes in the patient's health status, making early intervention more effective [18].

But the landscape is not complete, the Internet presents many blogs and digital opportunities for the patient to communicate about their own diseases [19]. Patients certainly need technical assistance regarding cure and services, but they also want to socialize, and they want to exchange experiences and knowledge with those who have the same problems [20, 21].

This is not a way to bypass clinicians, but it must be considered an important opportunity for acquiring information that is useful for people's care.

These opportunities foster the creation of new relationships, e.g., patient (family)-patient (family), patient (family)-social worker, and they encourage the creation of information, perhaps not technically medical, but surely useful for the patient's care and also for planning services.

The needs of the patient cannot be separated from those of their family; some-times the patient is not alone, and the family is an integral part of the care pathway. This aspect also needs to be taken into account for the care of the elderly and for care of the disabled population. When a patient is alone they are often helped by social workers and private charity agencies.

In all of these cases the relationships produce information that can be used for the care of people and for providing useful information for policy makers.

In this context the new medical models consider as positive the engagement of the patient in their own care process.

This concept, called "patient empowerment", has been described as the active participation of patients in their health and care pathway with the access, production, and use of information gained by using ICT tools.

Patient empowerment increases the patient's understanding of their disease, fosters health education and awareness of their own pathology, and allows direct contact with the professionals; all this exposes the risk of providing tools that support and improve self-management.

But this movement does not seem unstoppable; we can choose between nurturing the opportunities and fighting the model. Certainly we must pay attention: this concept encourages models of collaboration and they seem positive and useful, but we cannot foster the model of "do-it-yourself" health.

According to the opportunities offered by the concepts of patient empowerment, it seems worth noting the possibility for the patient to access their own medical records. We want to quote only one experience among many, i.e., the Open Note project, in which patients are invited to read their visit notes (compiled by doctors) through secure electronic patient portals. The aim of the project is to help to boost the quality of care and to make patients aware of their own health state [22]. "Open notes create partnerships toward better health and health care by giving everyone on the medical team, including the patient, access to the same information" says Tom Delbanco, MD, Beth Israel Deaconess Medical Center [22].

Against this background, different national or regional projects are proposing models related to patient engagement.

Such projects provide patients with access to and visualization of their own clinical data collected by professionals. The examples are many, and we can only mention some of them; for example, there are projects in Norway [23], Catalonia [24], Scotland [25], Czech Republic [26], France [27], Italy [28], and many others.

All the observations and experiences shown make us wonder what are the demands of patients and the demands of the "world connected to patients".

What emerges are the following concepts.

1. The patient's care must be considered unitary; even if the care pathway is fragmented, the clinical information must be amalgamated in order that the professionals (belonging to different organizations) can derive utility from this value-added model. People do not care if the clinical pathway is split up into individual work units, people care about their own health and ways of improving it; people are interested in the unity of their care. This implies that information referring to the patient must be centered on the patient and not centered on the different medical records.

   Patients need to have a strict relationship with their doctors, as well as with other ancillary professionals, such as nurses, and this is true also when new technologies are used. New technologies do not always turn the patient away from the doctor, sometimes they lead to an approach: "…[OpenNotes] gives me an opportunity to have a real good dialogue with my physician, to make sure that we're both on the same page…", a patient says (see the MyOpenNotes portal).

2. Patients need collaboration with other patients, social workers, and families of people suffering from the same disease. These relationships generate useful information about the needs of the patient and of their family. In these relationships, discomforts, problems, and tensions are expressed; they could be problematic for the relevant organizations or they could be a "cry for help", an alarm, a direction in which the ecosystem should look and cannot help but admit there is a need. The opportunity to share this information depends on the freedom of every individual and the desire to maintain some privacy. But we know that if this information is available (see the portals PatientLikeMe, 23AndMe), the clinical community and the whole ecosystem can obtain useful information [29]. So information produced by patients (in the form of sensations, problems, or their own notes on the pathology they are suffering) is a useful informative patrimony for the ecosystem.

3. The patient needs to be monitored frequently if they are suffering some chronic pathology. It is the mHealth world in which telemedicine devices can be used directly by patients; but not only the instruments are useful. If data can be shared and used, the knowledge of the health status of the patient grows for all the clinicians involved in the care process.

4. Patients need to know how to cope with their own pathology. They need to be educated to face their disease. They must know the environment of and the influences on their own pathology; in this way, they should be encouraged to improve. The tools for awareness, education, and improving are connected with the access to their own clinical information.

These concepts require more detailed elucidation.

Traditionally, clinical data are presented to patients as they are produced by the clinicians. With medical notes and referrals, the results of instrumental investigations are compiled by specialists for clinicians.

And these documents are presented to the patient, either in a face-to-face relationship or by the patient accessing these reports online.

In the first case, an explanation is possible (we have asserted that the presentation and explanation of clinical data or concepts are possible in the doctor-patient relationship), in the second case this is not always possible.

The fact remains that patients access clinical documents compiled by specialists for doctors.

The subject of access implies another important concept. It has been declared that medical notes referring to a patient are the property of the patient. This is true from a theoretical point of view. But a person exercises the right of property when they can make use of the object of the property. If the patient cannot understand the medical notes, what is the advantage that can result?

These arguments convince us that we need to rethink the way in which we present the online clinical data to the patients.

In a recent TedMed speech entitled "It's time to redesign medical data", Tomas Goetz affirmed [30]: "Your medical chart: it's hard to access, impossible to read – and full of information that could make you healthier if you just knew how to use it."

The challenge proposed by a health design organization [31, 32] had the aim of designing tools for presenting the patient's own medical records to the patient in order to make them more comprehensible.

The purpose of this challenge was to improve the design of medical records so that they would be more meaningful to and more usable by patients, their families, and others who take care of them. The following features were mooted: improving the visual layout and style of the information in the medical record, making it easier for patients to manage their health, enabling medical professionals to digest information more efficiently, and aiding caregivers, such as family members or friends, in their duties and responsibilities with respect to the patient.

The results have shown that improvements in medical strategies are possible. Such improvements include the possibility of ensuring total patient care, by coordinating and sharing accountability among multiple departments and providers, and preventing errors and the dissemination of misleading information by providing evidence-based clinical guidelines within medical strategies; the possibility of promoting and increasing patient participation by providing multiple convenient outlets for patient access to medical strategies; and the possibility of increasing patient independence with clear, well-organized, and optimal medical strategies.

At the end of this brief analysis we affirm that the value gained by including the patient in the ecosystem is information. Patients produce useful information for their own care, depending on their own needs. Information must be treated suitably so that it can offer the patients opportunities to use it in an appropriate manner. And we wonder whether the traditional medical records system can address these legitimate demands from the patients.

1.3.2   The Needs of Doctors and Researchers

Doctors are the main actors in the ecosystem.

They need to integrate the narrative produced in the encounter with the patient into useful clinical information.

As we have already said, this is not a simple action. In the doctor-patient relationship, doctors are attentive to signs and meanings and they use a code. During the encounter the dialog expresses the concepts that the doctor must incorporate in traditional database tables.

Very often the power of the narrative is lost, whereas different concepts are often hidden and they could be reused in the next encounters.

This concept is true for a GP who has the aim of knowing, over time, the health state of the patient; and it is broadened in the pathways of the new medical models. In these models each actor involved in the care process has the necessity of knowing the information produced in the different encounters of the workflow and each actor has the necessity of making available the information that the relationship produces during the encounter with the patient. The new medical models, as described above, are: precision medicine and system medicine, the network of pathologies, access to centers of medical excellence, the care of chronic disease, and cross-border care; all these can benefit from the concept of sharing clinical information.

In other words, what doctors need is the sharing of clinical information.

Very often this necessity for sharing is confused with the exchange of data. The two terms are very different and lead to the design and implementation of very different technical architectures. Data exchange presupposes deep knowledge of the semantics of the data, in which errors can induce misleading information; but the sharing of information allows access to data where and when it is necessary, directly by the actors who have acquired the information. Semantics, meaning, and correctness of information are saved, the information is reusable and the hidden knowledge can be extracted and treated.

From a social point of view, this is the concept of collaboration.

But there is another type of collaboration, which is expressed in the doctor-doctor relationship. In this relationship there is a simpler constraint on information in database tables, because the code used is generally comprehensible by the two actors. This collaboration happens, for example, in the event of a second opinion being sought, or during a consultation between specialists.

But also in this case the power of the narrative can be lost, even if the data discussed are well described.

Continuing to consider the events of collaboration between professionals, we can say that social networks for professionals are also platforms with sources of useful information; moreover, when the platforms allow mixed access (patients, professionals) the information is enriched and must be treated with suitable tools.

We also note that how to treat the complexity of clinical information is a need for precision medicine. In this case clinical information is combined with molecular data, environmental data, lifestyle information, and clinical information. The management of these different sources and different kinds of information is a great challenge for the sharing of information; not only is the usage of mathematical algorithms fundamental, such usage also implies collaboration between experts from different areas.

It is interesting to note that clinical research has deep connections with medical practice and with the patients' interactions.

Typically, clinical trials and clinical research projects produce ad hoc informatics tools for the management of data.

In such cases a huge amount of clinical information gained during clinical practice is not used, even if it were to be made available.

Currently clinical practice and medical research manage medical data on parallel planes, not taking advantage of the benefits offered by possible links. The reason for this is not just organizational, but also technological. Current middleware and frameworks for exchanging data must have ad hoc functions for exchanging the knowledge behind and beyond the data.

In this case also, researchers need collaboration, sharing information and suitable mathematical tools for extracting and managing information.

But we should not forget the chances offered by patient empowerment in this area [33]. Social platforms such as PatientLikeMe offer opportunities for the recruitment of patients and for exchanging data produced by patients. In the ecosystem the management of information for different aims cannot exclude any actor.

We have demonstrated, in regard to the relationships including doctors and researchers, that medical information is based on voluntary acts of encounter and on the publication, brokerage, and delivery of clinical information. The sources of information are data and the narrative, but considering only the power of the ecosystem and the opportunities offered by the sharing of information, it can be possible to respond to the requirements of the actors.

1.4   A Preliminary Discourse on the Architecture of the eHealth Ecosystem

From this brief analysis (there is still a lot to say and study) we can draw some conclusions of a technological character.

Currently two concepts regarding the infrastructure exist together: the universalist little governed, with few rules (short-ruled) idea regarding the Internet world and the monolithic integrationist governance of enterprise solutions. On completion of the monolithic solution, to exit from their own environment, enterprise solutions adopt the concept of "middleware" in order to create an integrated computing and communications platform, within an enterprise, built on the products of different suppliers with different systems.

The choice of either of these solutions, or a mixed solution, has important consequences for the technical functions to be implemented in the ecosystem.

For this reason the discourse on the architecture must be a priority.

Underlying the architectural discourse we find concepts of identification, addressing, routing, publication, and sharing, joined to business processes, capability, and capacity.

As we have described, the request of the ecosystem is that the context is a multiagency from an organizational point of view and highly collaborative from a social point of view, but the context in which intimate health problems are treated imposes the governance of the whole system. This is not a trivial problem, because, in reality, the universalist and monolithic solutions exist together, in which the first corresponds to an almost total absence of governance, while in the second case, the rules of each institution collide.

The point that overcomes the traditional architectures is the coordination across boundaries. This, in a federative context, involves the negotiation of shared meaning, purposes, and intentions rather than the imposition of central control and an obligation towards a direction. In practice, the federative architecture provides solutions with the intention of creating the possibility of more flexible, dynamic, and responsive distributions of the functionalities, and this also corresponds to a distribution of control and responsibility among agencies within communities [34].

These requirements clearly indicate that the topic here discussed principally regards governance and, as a clear implication of the analysis, governance and governability are, by nature, architectural.

Medical activity involves intention; as an intrinsic part of the cognitive process, we must include social interaction: intentionality and the relationships between intentions, actions, and outcomes lead to the provision of services.

This concept implies the inclusion of the social element in a system, i.e., it means that the system's components include people.

The challenge of complex care is therefore correlated with the coordination between different domains of existing functional centers, which must be able to maintain their respective identities, specializations, responsibilities, and relationships, including integration, but also must be able to participate in a dynamic integration around each user according to the needs of the situation, global policies, and principles of governance.

So we are thinking of a technical system in which a set of mutually interconnected components is provided. Together they exist in and interact with an environment. The relationship between such components is functional, in that the outputs of some functions form the inputs for others and the relationships between inputs and outputs follow one another and are created in different conditions. This description, at the technical level, creates, in some cases, complexity and in other cases, unpredictable behaviors in general.

From a functional point of view such a technical system corresponds to the composition of services. We have stressed that the so-called "longitudinal record" of a patient is a composition of different actions of relationships translated into clinical information, created in different situations by different actors (belonging also to different agencies), and that "pieces" of information can be composed in different ways in order to provide better care and in order to extract hidden information.

The composition of services becomes one of the most important functional requests.

This is because the applications for these contexts require a third and currently missing architectural solution, which is a federative component able to support the coordination of domains of specialism and integration that still hold their respective distinct identities and principles of governance, while they participate in some elements of common trust and coordination [35].

The requirements here go beyond the need for basic communication and the distribution of content and function that are provided by a universal infrastructure, to include also the basic functionalities we can identify as integration tools that overcome the traditional middleware.

We refer to three basic elements: portal functionality, switch element, and indexing object [36].

These basic elements, if well structured and composed, are the backbone of the federative platform.

Portal functionality. This is concerned with accessing, exchanging, and publishing content or other resources; the portal has the purpose of supporting the

publication and syndication mechanisms required to support catalogues and direc-
tories of offers and availabilities in the partnership.

Switch element. This is concerned with the routing, ordering, and coordination
of messages, transactions, and channels according to service processes and
workflows.

Indexing object. This represents the capability and consent to define which services (and users) can invoke which other services and service components in what
contexts.

To make explicit the basic functionalities and the other functionalities, we list the
following services.

Registration services, in which identities can be generated, allocated, and maintained and in which credentials can be issued. These may be the identities of people
(the actors in the ecosystem), but they can also be the identities of organizations (in
order to federate the federations), places, services (including the registration services themselves), physical devices, or publications.

Authentication services, which ensure a claimed identity against a register by
examining the presented credentials.

Index services, in which links between identities are registered and maintained.
Relationships are indexed in order to know who does what and with which device,
service, function, instrument, or tool. For example, this telemedicine device belongs
to Y, or this item of content was published by organisation Z as part of an ABC process. But also information W can be accessed by doctors X and H. Indexes are
important aspects of implementing consent policies and managing access, control,
distribution, and provenance in the sharing of information.

Workflow and transaction services. Workflow services are sometimes called
orchestration services (the term is derived from middleware theory) when what is to
be done is combined with aspects of where it will be done and by what means.
Workflow services allow the composition of "actions", allow the checking of activities, and define the transactions, i. e., the relationships between the actors.

Publication services, by which chunks of content registered in the network can
be made accessible to a target audience (individual, narrowcast, or broadcast).

Brokerage services, which connect user systems to a distributed set of local and
remote service systems.

Syndication services, for which registered content can be combined, organized,
and republished, preserving its original provenance. These services also allow content to be assembled and presented on the fly, in a federated network session. These
services, joined to an orchestration service, allow cataloguing to take place, involving the selection (possibly dynamic) and classification of published service offers
by information brokers for different types of users.

Mash-up services make up the work space of the users (the page of the portal, the
application, the apps) and consist of information collected on the fly according the
requests imposed by the clinical case treated.

Federative platforms can drive collaborative tools, allowing health interests and
medical knowledge to be shared, giving the actors a place to meet and share and
discuss their works, cases, interests, and their challenges, making health organizations more efficient and the networks of specialized interests a living place in which

knowledge is shared. This is the aim of the collaboration services; their purpose, according to the services for publication, syndication, and workflow, is to provide collaboration functions.

Services promoting collective intelligence finally collect a set of functions dedicated specifically to the management, delivery, and exploitation of the intelligence caught on the ecosystem. These functions correspond to the tools for extracting hidden information from the conversations and relationships; for treating molecular data; for joining molecular, environmental, and lifestyle data; and for managing huge amounts of information. The services, for example, provide tools and instruments for facilitating collaboration during precision medicine procedures, or they provide tools and instruments for producing complex clinical scenarios during a second-opinion session.

In more detail, the federated platform exposes a set of common components and it keeps the clinical information separate from the functions necessary for managing, storing, maintaining, treating, composing, and using it.

The term "common components" refers to a set of core informational elements and technical utilities that can be used by multiple applications.

Applications can use the components offered in the platform (from institutions, third parties, or software industries) according to the services logic and consistent with the medical workflow or functions of practice.

This approach facilitates the development of applications through shareable and reusable resources.

Information (including data and narrative, and—if necessary—ontologies and encodings) is kept separate from the functions generating it; this separation allows the composition of a single unit of information according to a sequence imposed by the immediate requests made by the clinicians from time to time, on the fly.

The reasons for maintaining applications separate from the components, and separating information from functions, correspond to a collaborative and open logic; this model allows the construction of collaborative applications able to share information, to compose knowledge, to create collaboration, to distribute knowledge, to join different sources of information, to extract knowledge by chunks of information, and to present the outcomes to different actors (including the patient) through different visual tools. Clinical information needed by the actors consists of a set of units of data, according to the requests made by those involved in the patient's care.

To summarize, the platform treats data and information. During the relationship, we must keep in mind the concept of narrative as comprehensive, but at the same time we must consider the functions necessary for managing the data (e.g., from instrumental investigations, blood tests, medical devices) in database tables. Data in this case is kept separate from the functions that originated it, in order to reuse the information [37]. Moreover, data is stored as a single unit with which the features that characterize it are associated.

These concepts regarding clinical information are strictly linked to the federative concept of the platform, in which information is treated as acts of relationships between actors belonging to different institutions, but with the desire to collaborate together; this collaboration is expressed through the publication, brokerage, and delivery of pieces of information composed together in order to provide care services.

Conclusions

Current medical records traditionally used in practice do not seem to be suited to the requirements of the new medical models, nor do they seem to be suited for the challenges in the health context imposed by the new concepts brought about by web2.0.

Rather than, ideally, dividing different records into diverse models corresponding to organizational purposes, each of which pretend to be the center, the focus of the design is shifted towards what counts and what are the needs of the actors, and this focus tends to consider the care of the patient as the true center.

We have therefore introduced the concepts of actors interacting with each other to create relationships that produce information.

The complex ecosystem is founded on voluntary acts of relationships between the actors that produce the clinical information; this is the value of the ecosystem.

Clinical information consists of "chunks" of information produced by different relationships (different actors in different agencies) through the coding of signs and meanings extracted by data and narrative.

The ecosystem we have described—in which the relationships among actors belonging to different organizations, institutions, and agencies are nurtured (continuing to express the actors' philosophy in the collaborative work that the medical job requires)—encourages the realization of federative platforms, in which clinical information and services are shared. This sort of sharing also fosters collaboration and the inclusion in the care workflow of all the actors, including the "empowered" patient.

The problem being treated so far cannot be addressed by the use of the classical enterprise approach, which consists of solutions that are directly integrated with proprietary mechanisms. In response to these challenges we propose to adopt a federative approach that supports and depends on trust and cooperation between agencies, allowing them to maintain their individual ethics, relationships with patients, and areas of responsibility and intervention. These agencies exchange information and coordinate actions in the interests of (and with the active participation and consent of) their shared clients. The rules, methods, and practices prescribed in the infrastructure system are an integral part of the use and governance of the supporting information and communications services.

References

1. Power to the patient: how mobile technology is transforming healthcare. A report from The Economist Intelligence Unit Limited 2015
2. Topol E (2015) The patient will see you now. The future of medicine is in your hands. Basic Books, New York. ISBN 978-0-465-05474-9
3. Toward Precision Medicine: Building a Knowledge Network for Biomedical Research and a New Taxonomy of Disease (2011) National Research Council (US) Committee on a framework for developing a new taxonomy of disease. National Academies Press (US), Washington, DC
4. Weston AD, Hood L (2004) Systems biology, proteomics, and the future of health care: toward predictive, preventative, and personalized medicine. J Proteome Res 3:179–196

5. Bar-Yam Y (2006) Improving the effectiveness of health care and public health: a multiscale complex systems analysis. Am J Public Health 96:459–466
6. Ahn AC, Tewari M, Poon CS, Phillips RS (2006) The clinical applications of a systems approach. PLoS Med 3(7):e209. doi:10.1371/journal.pmed.0030209
7. PCAST (President's Council of Advisors on Science and Technology) (2008) Priorities for personalized medicine. President's Council of Advisors on Science and Technology, September 2008 [online]. Available: http://www.whitehouse.gov/files/documents/ostp/PCAST/pcast_report_v2.pdf. Accessed 3 Aug 2011
8. Directive 2011/24/EU of the European Parliament and of the Council of 9 March 2011 on the application of patients' rights in cross-border healthcare
9. Rinaldi G, Gaddi A, Capello F (2013) Medical data, information economy and federative networks: the concepts underlying the comprehensive electronic clinical record framework. Nova Science Publishers, Hauppage, pp 11788–13619, p. 1–396. ISBN 978-1-62257-845-0
10. Barbieri M (2008) Biosemiotics: a new understanding of life. Naturwis-Senschaften 95(7):577–599, Springer 2008
11. Shannon CE (1948) A mathematical theory of communication. Bell Syst Tech J 27:379–423, 623–656, Luglio e Ottobre, 1948
12. Feynman RP (1959) Plenty of room at the bottom. Talk presented to the American Physical Society in Pasadena
13. Institute on Medicine (2001) Crossing the quality chasm: a new health system for the 21st century. Accessed 26 Oct 2015. http://iom.nationalacademies.org/Reports/2001/Crossing-the-Quality-Chasm-A-New-Health-System-for-the-21st-Century.aspx
14. Unifying Healthcare in Scotland (2015) Intersystems TrakCare case study. http://www.inter-systems.com/library/library-item/unifying-healthcare-in-scotland/. Accessed 26 Oct 2015
15. Cerner Corporation (2015) Accessed 26 Oct 2015. http://www.cerner.com/solutions/Hospitals_and_Health_Systems/
16. Eysenbach G (2008) Medicine 2.0: social networking, collaboration, participation, apomedia-tion, and openness. J Med Internet Res 10(3):e22, [on-line] available from: http://www.jmir.org/2008/3/e22/
17. Monteagudo JL, Moreno O (2007) Patient empowerment opportunities with eHealth, eHealth ERA report on priority topic cluster two and recommendations. Mar 2007. Available: http://ec.europa.eu/information_society/newsroom/cf/document.cfm?action=display&doc_id=320
18. Bos L, Marsh A, Carroll D, Gupta S, Rees M (2008) Patient 2.0 empowerment. In: Arabnia HR, Marsh A (eds) Proceedings of the 2008 international conference on semantic web & web services SWWS08, pp 164–167
19. Fox S, Jones S (2009) The social life of health information. Pew Internet & American Life Project, Washington, DC
20. Frost JH, Massagli MP (2008) Social uses of personal health information within PatientsLikeMe, an online patient community: what can happen when patients have access to one another's data. J Med Internet Res 10(3):e15
21. 23andMe (2015) [on-line] available from: https://www.23andme.com/. Accessed on 2015 Oct 29
22. http://www.myopennotes.org/. Accessed 25 Oct 2015
23. Patient's access to electronic health record. http://www.telemed.no/patients-access-to-electronic-health-record.5072035-247950.html. Accessed 29 Oct 2015
24. Garcia Cuyas F (2013) Health and ICT in Catalonia current situation and future plans. EHTEL. Barcelona, 12 Mar 2013
25. New Electronic Health Record rolls out across Scotland (2015) http://www.alliance-scotland.org.uk/news-and-events/news/2013/10/new-electronic-health-record-rolls-out-across-scotland/#.VjINHFUve00. Accessed 29 Oct 2015
26. Cabrnoch M, Hasić B (n.d.) Electronic health book—a unique Czech solution for eHealth. Health Technol 1(2–4) 57–69. doi:10.1007/s12553-011-0006-z
27. de Lusignan S, Seroussi B (2013) A comparison of English and French approaches to provid-ing patients access to summary care records: scope, consent, cost. Stud Health Technol Inform 186:61–65

28. Ministero della Salute (2010) Il Fascicolo Sanitario Elettronico. Linee Guida Nazionali. Roma, 11 Nov 2010
29. Wicks P, Keininger DL, Massagli P, de la Loge C, Brownstein C, Isojärvi J, Heywood J (2012) Perceived benefits of sharing health data between people with epilepsy on an online platform. Epilepsy Behav 23(1):16–23
30. TedMed (2010) Filmed October 2010. https://www.ted.com/talks/thomas_goetz_it_s_time_to_redesign_medical_data
31. http://healthdesign.devpost.com/
32. http://healthdesignchallenge.com/
33. http://partners.patientslikeme.com/products-and-services/patient-recruiting/clinical-trial-awareness. Accessed on 25 Oct 2015
34. Garrety K, McLoughlin I, Wilson R, Zelle G, Martin M (2014) National electronic health records and the digital disruption of moral orders. Soc Sci Med 101:70–77
35. McLoughlin I, Wilson R, Martin M (2013) Digital government at work: a social informatics perspective. Oxford University Press, Oxford
36. Rinaldi G, Martin M, Gaddi A (2011) Establishing an infrastructure for tele-care: combining the socio-technical and the clinical. In: Bos L, Dumay A, Goldschmidt L, Verhenneman G, Yogesan K (eds) Handbook of digital homecare. Berlin, Springer
37. Baele T (2002) Archetypes: constraint-based domain models for future-proof information systems. In: Workshop on behavioural semantics (OOPSLA'02).

An Infrastructural Approach to Clinical Information

2

Mike Martin

2.1   What Is the Problem?

The title of this volume refers to "new perspectives" on electronic health records, but it must be recognised that, in the development of the information infrastructure to support clinical care, novelty is usually both relative and local and that in the last quarter of a century progress has been slow and rather fragmented. In this chapter, I would like to revisit an approach to supporting clinical recording and the exchange and use of clinical information which was first developed around 2000 but which was ignored in the context of the subsequent Connecting for Health (CfH) programme of 2003–2010 in the English NHS. That programme adopted a top-down, integrationist approach which attempted to deploy national applications to address the needs of health records and service management. The alternative approach we will consider here is best described as infrastructural, and it stands in marked contrast to the structural or applications-oriented approaches which continue to dominate the health-care market. This dominance is maintained by two powerful forces. The first of these is the interest of both the software systems supply sector and public sector procurement systems to put concrete, well-defined offers at the centre of the business model and customer relationship whether this is applied in the large organisational context of acute care or of provision at the national or regional levels or to the smaller-scale supply relationships which may prevail in primary care. Even though, in the latter case, the approach has been much more user and clinician centred and has, as a result, had greater clinical success, retaining ownership of the architecture of a clearly defined product or service package and platform remains a high commercial priority for systems suppliers and represents a necessary simplification for procurers.

M. Martin
Newcastle University Business School, Newcastle University, Newcastle, UK
e-mail: mike.martin@newcastle.ac.uk

© Springer International Publishing Switzerland 2017
G. Rinaldi (ed.), *New Perspectives in Medical Records*, TELe-Health,
DOI 10.1007/978-3-319-28661-7_2

The second force which is maintaining the structural, applications-oriented approach to clinical record systems is the dominance of concrete thinking in the way that clinicians and health-care managers define and pursue their needs and objectives. Abstraction is not a tool that figures significantly in the way that clinicians are trained to think; they are required, for very good reasons, to focus on the specifics of concrete presentations. In this mindset, it becomes very difficult to think of an electronic clinical record as anything other than a physical software application presented through a concrete user interface and to evaluate it purely in terms of the functionality of that interface, the underlying data structures that are incorporated and their relationship to specific clinical (and service provision) work and contexts.

It is clear, then, that proposing an infrastructural approach, in this context, represents a challenge to the prevailing culture which is likely to evoke incomprehension and rejection. This is the inevitable consequence of a failure to achieve any real engagement. An absolute prerequisite for such engagement is a very careful and explicit approach to defining and discussing an architectural terminology and exploring the precise levels of abstraction at which specific terms are being used. But the caveat remains: the move from conventional conceptions and language to this new one requires effort and commitment which is usually only generated as the result of a recognition that the current approaches have become significantly problematic. The area in which this realisation is becoming most apparent and acute is that of complex long-term conditions involving care close to home and in the community. This is the context in which primary care is situated with additional demands for coordinated, multi-agency and multidisciplinary responses from other clinical and non-clinical actors. Power and influence in the clinical domain, however, tend to reside in the acute specialisms in the tertiary sector, and this creates a third component which tends to maintain the status quo in the delivery of health informatics.

Before considering the term "infrastructure" and how it can be applied to clinical information, we will first consider another term which I have already used; this is "architecture". In the paragraph above, I used it in the conventional sense of the high level technical design of a product or service which is presumed to be the intellectual property of a supplier. This meaning, however, belies the etymology of the word: "arche" refers to two possible meanings, before or prior, as in archaeology, or chief and leading as in "archbishop". "Techne" also has two meanings: the exercise of skill and the performance of technical work on the one hand or material or matter[1] on the other. So, the term has a quite rich set of meaning including that of the chief or leading technical work, but also to the work that precedes any technical work. We are particularly concerned with this latter meaning of architecture in this chapter.

When we apply this concept of architecture to the ways we enable and support the recording and exchange of clinical information, we must recognise that there are many different "technes" to be considered. These include not only medical, nursing and allied professional work but also care coordination and service brokerage, management and planning, education, research, development, informatics and

---

[1] Consider tectonics, for example.

communication system design work. We must also consider the technicalities of being a patient, particularly one with a complex long-term condition and multiple co-morbidities. From this perspective, the means by which these different perspectives can communicate with each other is an important aspect of architecture.

This wide and heterogeneous variety of needs and constraints represents a fundamental challenge to the applications-oriented approach which represents an attempt to design a unified response which will satisfy all of them. Faced with the inevitable failure to achieve such unity and integration in a single product, the problem is transformed into an equally intractable one of achieving "interworking" and "information sharing" between heterogeneous products and their users, where technical systems suppliers' interests are clearly to maximise and preserve the sales potential associated with the needs to interwork, making this a significant aspect of the cost of ownership and use of their products. While concepts such as open source and ever more inclusive and comprehensive data and document standards are pursued in the face of this impasse, I want to suggest that the problem is deeper but, in some senses, simpler than this.

The diagnosis here is that of an absence of architecture, in the sense we have defined it. It is the lack of a framework in which all of these different technical domains can engage in effective mutual conversations, not only about the nature of the technical systems, standards and facilities they need to do their respective jobs but also to coordinate their ongoing conversations and relationships which constitute the delivery, governance, innovation and learning of the community of care itself.

In this chapter we will explore an outline of such a framework. This is not offering a new or competing design of a product or a platform: that would be adopting the traditional meaning of "architecture" which we must regard as part of the problem. Rather it is a different approach to conceptualising and talking about these issues and the way we are responding to them. My claim is that a key element in making progress is to reframe them in terms of infrastructure and the relationships between information infrastructure; structural operation, which, in this case, is the delivery of care and well-being services; and the governance of service processes and relationships.

In the next section, I will briefly describe the Durham and Darlington EHR demonstrator as an example of an infrastructural approach. This represented a model of a shared electronic record within a care community. The characteristic of the model was that the record, as such, was a side effect or by-product of clinical communications supported by a messaging and publication infrastructure. The following sections will then elaborate some of the architectural theories that underpin and justify this approach.

2.2   The EHR Demonstrator

The Durham and Darlington EHR prototype was based on a clinical scenario in coronary care; at its core was a sequence of clinical messages concerning an imaginary patient. Examples of these are summarised in Fig. 2.1.

- Registrations
- Prescription 1
- Consent registration
- GP Publication
- GP eczema
- Referral to Cardiologist
- Radiology Referral
- Lab Orders
- Cardio Appointment
- Radiology Appointment
- Lab Results

- ECG Result
- CXR Result
- Ambulance Call
- Ambulance Results
- A&E Triage
- A&E Orders
- A&E Radiology
- A&E Rad Results
- A&E Lab Results
- Hospital Discharge
- Referral for Exercise Test

Fig. 2.1 Simulator messages and transactions

Each message was implemented through standard XML schema and a publication rule which defined what data would be extracted from the message, where it would be recorded and how a root publication server would be notified. The specific configuration of these rules was seen as the consequence of "joint acts of publication and consent" by a clinician and a patient as a part of the pathway definitions of the clinical situation.

The project had developed a set of architectural models of both physical systems, the processes they supported and also the intentional aspects of the roles and conversations that were being enacted. Some of these will be explored later in this chapter. One of the outcomes was the ability to define the set of systems and information services and a reference network configuration that would support a local community of care and its health economy. This community was represented as a federation of member agencies rather than as the functional components of an integrated, monolithic enterprise. This is seen in the right-hand pane of the EHR demonstrator dashboard shown in Fig. 2.2 which represents three layers between source systems and user systems, both of which represent existing health and social care systems operated by the members of the health community. The new elements are publication systems, hub systems and gateway or access systems which together represent an extendable federated infrastructural network.

The other panes in this prototype application contain the list of messages in the system (the timeline) and the current message being processed in the simulation sequence.

As messages were played through the demonstrator, their passage through the network between servers and applications was visualised on the system map, and the consequences on the content of the EHR, in the browser window represented in Fig. 2.3, were updated. At each stage, as the events unfolded, the prototype shared record could be evaluated for clinical relevance and completeness.

This rapid prototype was constructed in a few weeks by a single programmer under the guidance of the clinical and technical directors of the project. When the projects' main technical team saw it, their reaction was that they had thought they were involved in a database project and that the issues were data selection, coding and cleansing with the creation of new mappings and canonical forms – processes

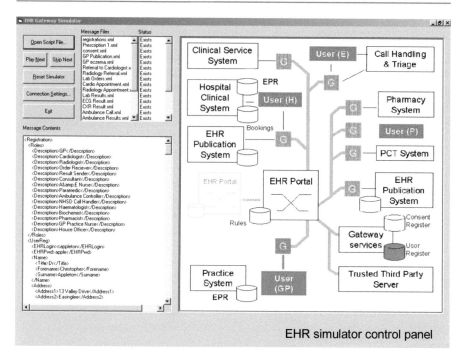

Fig. 2.2 This simulator dashboard shows clinical messages passing between network nodes and being captured in publication servers

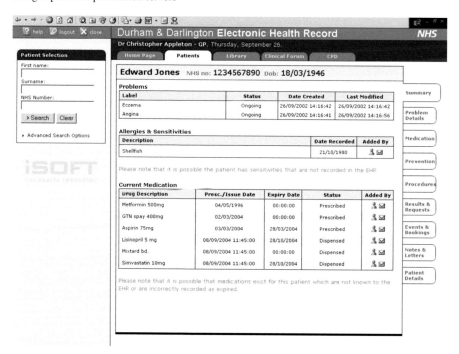

Fig. 2.3 The resulting patient record in which each entry could be traced back to its origin in a clinical message

that had proved extremely troublesome and had not succeeded. Now, they said, they realised that the problem was really one of message and transaction management. The clinical representatives who evaluated the content against the requirements of the clinical scenario judged that the apparently live, evolving record was adequate and appropriate and that a high reliance could be put on the quality of the data because, if they needed, they could verify, by drilling down on any item of information, that it had come from specific real transactions rather than been collected for the purposes of a recording system.

They then commenced discussions on the design of clinical messages and whether this or that item of data could or should be included and/or published to the record. It was also clear in these discussions that this shared record was not seen as a substitute for existing primary or acute records, with their clusters of local and specific contexts and purposes. Rather it was seen as a valuable supporting and integrating tool. Note that nobody made explicit entries into the shared record; its content was a side effect of external messaging events and transactions. The project did not have the resources to examine the practical consequences of the support of service management and secondary uses although these issues were considered at the architectural level.

These results were of course preliminary and only indicative; it was clear that many issues still required resolution. However, language and attitudes in the locally engaged community had changed, and this included clinical users, service and strategic management and the technical developers from the systems supplier. The discourse of data quality, security, access control and ownership, which had dominated much of the discussions on "data sharing" up to that point, changed to ones of governance responsibilities and needs to know or to clinically inform. All of the content of the "record" had already been shared and had an explicit purpose or set of purposes because it came from the content of structured messages that had already been sent and received. The contexts and provenance of each item of data had been preserved because it could be traced back to the message context, sender and role in which it originated, that is to say, to a specific type of conversation. At the same time, the "record" was not merely a collection of original documents but could be organised and filtered to meet the requirements of specific roles, contexts and use sessions.

As indicated above, this work was overtaken by events and did not come to fruition. It is not offered as a blueprint or plan but as a provocation to thought. In the next section, we examine the thinking that lays behind the demonstrator we have described.

2.3   What Is Information Infrastructure?

We have characterised the approach we have described as "infrastructural", but this is a term that is used in many distinct disciplinary settings and has many corresponding meanings which are related, but are not identical. Two key aspects of the term, as we are using it here, are:

1. It represents a standardised and reusable resource and capacity which supports multiple instances of some more or less standardised type of activity for a community of users.

2. There are degrees of freedom in the detail of the supported activity which leaves room for innovation in use. This is in contrast to the applications-oriented approach which intends to support only the mandated use cases, business processes and logics.

Clinical communications take many different forms in different contexts, but there is a core set of requirements which differentiate them from, for example, commercial or social conversations, transactions and relationships. The problem of abstraction we face is to be precise and accurate about what these core commonalities are so that they can be supported by the infrastructure while preserving the required flexibilities for appropriation and adaptation to specific local needs, in this case, the many different clinical messages and transactions that take place within and across a care community. We will now explore a simple model of clinical communication or, more precisely, clinical "conversation". The distinction we are making is that we are not only considering processes, things that people do, but we are also concerned with their purposes and intentions. So, our diagram will depict what we will call "acts" represented as blue arrows and "instruments" which are labelled lozenges. As we will see, there may be a range of corresponding real-world actions which may represent an appropriate performance of the intended acts.

2.4 Clinical Communication

It is a constitutive principle in clinical contexts that any act performed by a clinician in respect of a patient should be performed under the informed consent of that patient. The clinical act we will consider, as an example, is a referral by a GP (the generator) of a patient (the subject) to a hospital specialist (the interpreter). The notion of informed consent entails a new role and responsibility, that of councillor and a new instrument which is taken to be an explanation. This responsibility may, of course, be combined with and seen as part of generation, or it could be allocated to a third party: the GP explains or the practice nurse explains in a separate encounter and conversation.

As we have indicated, the model represents the problem, not the solution. Subsequent design options could be the proposal that the explanation takes the form of:

(a) Ten-minute discussion about the contents of a relevant brochure by the generator/councillor, which was designed for the purpose and which the patient then takes away
(b) A suggestion that the patient looks up a URL
(c) An assumption that the patient understands and that further explanation is superfluous

The response to the explanation is the granting, or withholding, of consent. This involves an act by the subject on, or with, another instrument. This again may take a number of different forms both explicit and implicit:

A signature on a document or a tick in a screen as part of an authenticated session

A verbal statement which is noted in the record by the recipient (in this case our
   generator role)
The absence of any verbal statement or indication, taken to be implied consent

So, in our intentional model, we represent the problem or requirement, and
any suggestion of a way of implementing it invites the question "do we accept
this to mean that?" Intentional, conversational models provide a bridge
between:

(a) Statements of policy which are, necessarily, rhetorical texts requiring interpre-
    tation, concerned with feelings and attitudes, such as trustworthiness and safety,
    as well as concrete things such as rules
(b) Representations of a distribution of roles and responsibilities in a set of conver-
    sations and the instruments that will signify the implied information exchanges
    and the transactional acts

We can continue our policy and intentionality analysis of clinical communication by the consideration of records and recording. It is a second principle of clinical action that any significant clinical act must be entered into a record; this is
considered an essential part of clinical governance and of clinical care responsibilities. The generation of a record produces a new responsibility of custodianship
of that record. This is the duty to ensure that any future use of the information is
in accordance with the consent and purposes of the original generation. Thus, we
see a new set of future interpreters of the record, and we represent the relationship
between them and the original subject at the future date when the record is
accessed.

A final remark in Fig. 2.4 is that, since the communication takes place across a
boundary of governance, in this case between a practice and a hospital, there is a
logical requirement for recording and custodianship in both of the domains. This
raises the issue about the contexts and purposes on the interpretation of records in
these two domains and whether a single record, held in common, is adequate or
appropriate. Clearly there are some elements of clinical record which are generic
and shared because they represent the relationship of the subject with the national
service or are concerned with the subject as such rather than to any particular aspect
of the particular clinical relationship. Other aspects of the record are specific to each
of the domains and to the particular care relationships. These subtleties of conversation and relationship bring into question the simplistic notion of the integrationist
approach that asserts that a single shared record results in "integrated" care. It
underlines the fact that clinical care is not delivered in a single domain but has multiple contexts.

The key methodological steps behind the infrastructural approach adopted in the
DDEHR project were:

(a) Clinical communications have the conversational implications represented in
    Fig. 2.4, and their electronic support must both respect and reflect this.

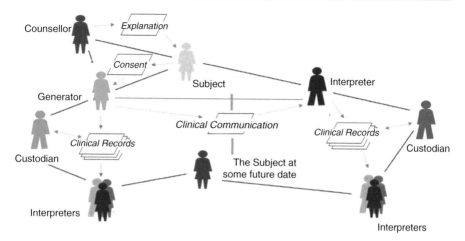

Fig. 2.4 Clinical communication as a set of roles and conversational relationships over time and space

(b) Care pathways and health-care journeys are composed of sequences and networks of these conversations and represent the contexts in which information is generated and interpreted.

(c) The electronic platform should support these conversations and maintain the links between them.

This final step is important. It amounts to asking, in each instance of generation of information within any clinical conversation, are there other contexts, i.e. future conversations, which we would want to inform or which needs to know about this? We could describe this as an examination of the "conversations between conversations". The shared record infrastructure then provides the means for delivering this information on the occasions and in the contexts which are intended.

The clinicians who examined and evaluated the DDEHR demonstrator asserted that they did not see the shared electronic record as a substitute for their own professional records but as a supporting tool which relieved them of many of the mud-line recording tasks and provided them with the means to coordinate and to ensure the continuing care of their patients.

2.5   Conclusions and Observations

In this chapter I have only been able to give the briefest of outlines of an architectural discourse of an infrastructural approach. I would stress that this does not represent new technologies or new design but is at least the beginnings of a new way of talking about both the challenges and needs of care and the structures and supporting services required to govern its delivery.

The original project took place 15 or more years ago, and it is interesting to note that there have been a number of developments since then that adopt different aspects of the infrastructural and, as a consequence, federalist as opposed to integrationist approach that has been described. Possibly the clearest examples of this is the document federation approach of the XDS Affinity Domain and the Integrated Health Environment (IHE) standards and designs.

However, the core message that I am trying to give is a methodological one. Modelling requirements in terms of functions using such tools as use cases and workflows has proved adequate in the world of commerce and of industry. Here, there is little or no ambiguity: the intention is simple – to stay in business and to earn profits within a regulatory framework. Health and Social Care is more complex because there is ambiguity and emergence which is irreducible. Attempts to reduce relational services of well-being and development to the mechanisms of business processes have tended to result not in systems of care but of box ticking and target gaming which has, in turn, resulted in neglect and abuse.

The need for systematic rigour remains, however, and systems have to be engineered. I have tried to indicate an approach to this new level of rigour which involves abstracting and modelling intentionality through the concept of a clinical conversation and showing how such a model can underpin an infrastructural approach in which the record that needs to be shared is generated and maintained as a consequence or side effect of clinical messaging and transaction.

Acknowledgement The author would like to acknowledge the contribution of colleagues in the DDEHR project particularly that of Dr Nick Booth who was the Clinical Director.

Suggested Reading

1. Greenhalgh T, Potts HW, Wong G, Bark P, Swinglehurst D (2009) Tensions and paradoxes in electronic patient record research: a systematic literature review using the meta-narrative method. Milbank Q. 87(4):729–88
2. http://eprints.ucl.ac.uk/18821/1/18821.pdf
3. Eason K (2007) Local sociotechnical system development in the NHS National Programme for Information Technology. J Inf Technol. 22:257. doi:10.1057/palgrave.jit.2000101

From Big Data to Big Insights: The Role of Platforms in Healthcare IT

3

Alberto Di Meglio and Marco Manca

3.1   Introduction

During history scientific research has gone through a series of critical shifts. It started with empirical observation and description of natural phenomena in ancient civilisations until the adoption of the experimental method in the sixteenth century (empirical and experimental research). It moved from the formal elaboration of mathematical principles (theoretical research) to the adoption of computer-generated simulation to solve increasingly complex models (computational research). At the end of the twentieth century, the increasing amount of experimental data and simulation has given rise to a new shift whereby experiments, models and simulations are combined into large-scale scientific research projects across the world (eScience) [1].

In the past several years, scientific research has seen a dramatic rise in the amount and rate of production of data collected by instruments, detectors or sensors. The LHC detectors at CERN produce a staggering 1 PB of data per second, a figure bound to increase during the second LHC run started in 2015. Large research infrastructures are deployed by international and European organisations like CERN, ESA or EMBL in Europe or the NSF in the USA or initiatives like EGI and ELIXIR in Europe or OSG or XSEDE in the USA. These research infrastructures are expected to produce increasingly large amounts of data in diverse scientific domains, such as physics, meteorology, neurology, genetics or radio astronomy, produced by satellite imaging devices, high-performance genomic sequencers, neutron diffractometers, x-ray antennas or particle detectors.

The increasingly ubiquitous use of smartphones, fitness trackers and many other types of connectable, portable or wearable devices generates unprecedented amounts of data with the so far unexploited potential for scientific, industrial, commercial and

A. Di Meglio (✉) • M. Manca
Department of Information Technology, CERN, Geneva, Switzerland
e-mail: alberto.di.meglio@cern.ch

© Springer International Publishing Switzerland 2017
G. Rinaldi (ed.), *New Perspectives in Medical Records*, TELe-Health,
DOI 10.1007/978-3-319-28661-7_3

public organisation use but also concerning impact on privacy and confidentiality of personal information.

The use of big data methods in biomedical applications is still in its infancy. The interest typically comes from two main areas, genomic-driven research and the increasing use of electronic health records and their application to the provision of medical or insurance services to patients. In between lies a vast array of potentially disruptive applications in research, clinical or translational medicine and person-alised services.

One of the big hurdles to overcome is the relative lack of maturity and the com-plexity of most of the tools and methods required to harness large enough datasets and extract nuggets of value from a landfill of very noisy data in often incompatible formats. In addition, in the specific context of medical applications, the interest in big data is expected to appear at the "local" level rather than at a centralised level. Relating small subgroups of data of interest to the deluge of global data is currently not obvious and might require explicit support from tools and methodologies.

In this chapter, we present a general definition of big data and a simplified, but comprehensive, value delivery model based on the concepts of services and plat-forms. The model presented emphasises the separation of roles and responsibilities across different technology and service layers and aims at clarifying and simplify-ing the implementation of big data infrastructures, tools and applications focusing on end users' functional requirements in a way that could be profitably used by healthcare researchers and practitioners.

3.2   What Is Big Data?

The term big data is used to indicate in a rather generic way unspecified, but sub-stantially large datasets. The perceived size of big data is usually relative to the technology available to acquire, store, analyse, curate or preserve the data and can even vary across different communities of use at any given time. The now tradi-tional way of defining the concept of big data is by describing its properties. The original description was proposed by Doug Laney in a 2001 research report by Gartner [2]. The model describes big data in terms of its *volume* (the quantity of data), its *velocity* (the speed at which data is produced) and its *variety* (the many different types of data sources and formats). The model is known as the *3Vs* model.

After the initial orderly and somewhat controlled scientific applications of big data started moving to real-world scenarios, the idea of collecting huge amounts of data as a potential panacea for many complex problems emerged, albeit not always with clear purposes and "contracts" among the different stakeholders. As a conse-quence, the original model was further extended with additional properties, describ-ing other aspects of big data, more related to quality and value than physical properties. A popular set of additional properties today includes *variability*, which describes the fact that data quantities, rates and formats can change, sometimes in unforeseeable and inconsistent ways; *veracity*, which refers, for example, to the qual-ity of the generated data, the difficulty of capturing accurate provenance information or the often low signal-to-noise ratio; and *value*, which highlights, very significantly, the hidden, but potentially high, value that can be produced by properly managing and processing the data.

The notion of value is of course strongly related to the purpose for which data is captured and processed and can arbitrarily refer to increased knowledge, better end user services, more efficiency, economical value or any other type of benefit depending on the context.

3.3   Large-Scale Service Platforms

The Vs model is a useful way of qualitatively, if not quantitatively, capturing the specific aspects of what distinguishes traditional data from big data. However, it does not provide per se any indication of how very large quantities of rapidly generated, inhomogeneous, inconsistent, noisy data can be actually acted upon to produce value.

In order to understand big data, a model must be provided to define what is required to capture, store, process, distribute or visualise data and generate information and knowledge. A possible model can be constructed by considering the different processes, functions and technologies that a big data management system must include to go from the physical world from which raw data is generated to the actual production of valuable information.

The basic function is provided by the technologies necessary to generate data. As introduced in the previous section, data is generated by a great variety of devices, sensors and detectors, in hundreds of different formats and at different speeds. A typical hospital facility can produce hundreds of gigabytes of data per day from PET or MRI imaging devices, laboratory tests, ECGs, prescriptions, patient records and more; hundreds of millions of wearable devices produce several megabytes of data per person per day each; modern high-speed genomic sequencers can produce tens of terabytes of data in a few hours; the Australian Square Kilometre Array Pathfinder (ASKAP) radio telescope streams almost 3 gigabytes of data per second; the Large Hadron Collider (LHC) experiment detectors produce today a combined data rate of the order of 1 petabyte per second; and so on.

Once the data is produced, it can be stored and processed in place, but most of the time it must be distributed to other storage or processing facilities across wide-area infrastructures. Sustained transfer of large quantities of data has been for one of the major challenge in the construction of distributed data networks. The high energy physics started addressing this problem in the early years of the twenty-first century, deploying dedicated high-bandwidth fibre-optics networks and connecting them across continents. Today, with the advent of social networks and on-demand media content streaming, the problem is largely solved from a technology point of view. However, if scientific research infrastructures were at the forefront of the technology until 5–10 years ago, consumer industry has taken the lead today. Concepts as Content Delivery Networks (CDN) [3] and Named Data Networking (NDN) [4] are not extensively applied to research infrastructures. In addition, when large data transfers must occur across geographically distributed sites, better ways of rapidly configuring the network paths and avoiding bottlenecks are called for. Technology and standards that promise to address these requirements, like Software-Defined Networking (SDN) [5] implementations, are emerging and are increasingly being adopted by network equipment providers.

Storage of increasingly large amounts of data and efficient long-term archival and retrieval is another important function of distributed big data architectures. Storage media technology is rapidly evolving to address big data requirements, but it is still difficult to design storage systems able to provide configurable quality of service for such diverse applications as real-time data streaming, offline processing or long-term preservation. Increasingly larger-sized SSD discs promise to help storing huge volumes of data in compact formats, but efficient ways of filtering, structuring and compressing the data must also be applied to prevent unnecessary and costly waste of space.

Once raw data is available either as a more or less continuous stream or stored in suitably large storage systems, the next step to start turning data into information is by processing it to find insights and correlations or to build models. Additionally, theoretical models can be simulated to produce additional data used to predict how physical systems might work under specified conditions and constraints. Several different computing architectures can be used from local batch systems or clusters to distributed grid, cloud or volunteer computing infrastructures to powerful high-performance computing systems. However, a major problem with data processing and simulation today lies in the fact that the software must be often optimised to run on specialised computing platforms like multicore or many-core CPUs or GPUs and special programming skills are needed to produce such software.

Data can be processed in different ways and for different purposes, but a paradigm that fits well with the goal of extracting value from large quantities of data is *data analytics* or the process of identifying meaningful patterns from seemingly random data. Although data analytics is far from being a new concept [6], it has emerged in recent years as a useful tool for business intelligence, financial modelling and forecast, optimisation of industrial processes and other disciplines where large quantities of inhomogeneous data need to be processed. Several open-source systems exist today, like the paradigmatically famous Hadoop, which has been designed specifically to store and process large quantities of data using programming models like MapReduce by means of parallel, distributed algorithms on large computing clusters [7].

When dealing with large quantities of seemingly incoherent data possibly coming from different sources in different formats, finding useful patterns or models is not trivial. Additionally, if the goal is to define models that not only fit the available data but provide useful insights to predict future behaviours, then sophisticated methods are required. The application of techniques from machine learning or natural language processing to big data has become a field of great interest for many applications, but requires multidisciplinary skills not easy to find especially when they have to be combined with at least general knowledge of the subject matter, like medical research, clinical trials or diagnostics. Additionally, in applications where

Fig. 3.1 The typical service-oriented architecture

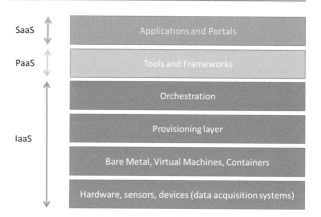

the multidisciplinary skill sets become critical, as is the case in many medical research applications, the advantage of machine learning over more traditional techniques based on abstract thinking or semantic analysis is still unproven.

At the end of the process outlined so far, the data has been transformed into information, by adding additional data, or metadata, that contextualise the raw numbers for specific purposes and applications. However, since a standard human being cannot immediately grasp the meaning of data or information presented in basic numeric form, intuitive, yet sophisticated, ways of visualising and manipulating information are required. Software applications able to work with this type of distributed, data-driven scenarios are also necessary, especially if the objective is to use the generated information in real-time situations across different types of wide-area and mobile networks. Once all this is available and we can measure the benefit produced by using data, we can say that value has been produced.

3.4   Service-Oriented Architectures and the "As-a-Service" Model

Dealing with the technical aspects of many of the functional components described so far requires specific knowledge and competencies that cannot anymore be found in individual, no matter how bright, scientists or practitioners. In order to enable correct implementation and exploitation of the value-generating functional chains, a specialisation is required. The components briefly described so far can be further classified in at least three main categories or layers (Fig. 3.1):

- *Infrastructures*: this layer includes all components used to capture, transfer, store and process data, such as data acquisition systems and devices, networks, storage systems and computing platforms and infrastructures. This layer must mainly address aspects related to volume and velocity, but it can often be considered neutral in terms of variety, variability or veracity, and value is still hidden at this point.

- *Platforms*: this layer includes the data processing tools making use of the infrastructure layer to derive information from data, produce generalised models, apply the models and make estimates and predictions. This layer must be able to cope with the aspects of volume, velocity and variability and must address veracity. This is where the signal-to-noise ratio is increased and valuable information takes shape.
- *Software* (*or applications*): this layer includes the end user facing applications to interact with the systems, upload and download data and information, visualise the data, create reports, etc. This layer is in principle less affected by volume or variability, since filtering and reduction have already happened and veracity should have already been assessed. It must therefore address aspects of variability (formats) and value. This is where the information can actually be exploited.

Each layer should come with well-defined roles and responsibilities, expertise, quality of service agreements and interfaces and should interoperate as part of a general service-oriented architecture (SOA). A popular model to define such boundaries is the "As-a-Service" model, whereby each layer is managed by specialised entities providing access to sets of defined services and quality levels without the need for the user to know how to implement the underlying technology. In the context of this model, typical layers are defined, such as *IaaS* (Infrastructure-as-a-Service), *PaaS* (Platform-as-a-Service), *SaaS* (Software-as-a-Service) or even *Information-as-a-Service* or *DaaS* (Data-as-a-Service).

3.5   State of the Art of the Service Layers

It is worth taking a closer look at some of the services briefly described above, since an understanding of what is currently available and a correct definition of expectation are crucial for the success of a project, especially in medical research where data can really fall in all the Vs of the extended Vs model.[1]

3.5.1   Data Comes in Many Different Sizes and Types

Data is of course at the centre of architecture. A thorough understanding of the data used and generated in a project is a fundamental element of its success. No technology can help with a poor understanding of the end goal of the activity and the constraints dictated by the data before, during and after the project or activity is completed.

Beyond the generic properties defined by the big data Vs model, data has a relatively large variety of additional qualities. It is, for example, necessary to classify

---

[1] As a comparison, consider that, for example, in high energy physics, although volume and velocity are important parameters, variety is actually quite limited and variability is easy to predict or control.

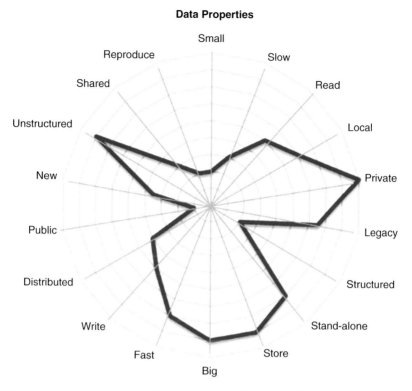

Fig. 3.2   An example of how to classify data in a project. Different projects have different requirements and the computing, storage and analysis platform must support such requirements. A clear understanding of the data is the starting point in the design of the computing infrastructure

data also based on aspects of expected use, locality, format, distribution constraints, etc. Fig. 3.2 exemplifies a possible way of understanding the relative importance of several data properties in a project as a preliminary step to the design of a suitable service architecture.

A useful classification should include at least the properties in Table 3.1.

3.5.2   Computing Systems

Computing platforms provide the functionality to execute calculations (process) of the data to transform it or produce additional data. There are two aspects to consider, the actual processing units (CPU) and the way the processing units are organised in order to receive and process data and generate the results or computing infrastructures.

Even if we only consider commodity computing systems, the evolution of the technology in the past 20 years has been quite interesting. Until the beginning of the year 2000, Moore's law could empirically ensure that software designed for a family of

Table 3.1 Classification of data properties

Size	Small → big	The amount of data, metadata and information produced by the acquisition systems, simulation, processing, etc. It is relative to the size and duration of the project/activity and available technology, but today big means not less than several 10 s of TB over a short period of time (hours or days)
Rate	Slow → fast	The rate at which data is generated and processed relative to the usage requirements of the project. It is fast, for example, if many GB or TB of data are generated over short periods of time and must be analysed in real time
I/O	Read → write	Is the data typically written once and read many times or by many users? Or is it made of many small files that have to be combined, read once and discarded?
Locality	Local → distributed	Where is the data? Is it available and processed in a single data centre or does it come from many different sources?
Confidentiality	Private → public	Who can access the data? Does it have to be restricted?
Age	Legacy → new	Is the data already available? In which formats? Is it generated by the project? Are the tools to read/process is still available? For how long must it be maintained?
Form	Structured → unstructured	Is the data encoded in typical database-like formats with predefined tags and associated meaning? Or is it made of free text or images? Is this one of the most stereotyped properties of big data? Can we access the hidden value of free-format data? How do we interpret it in a way that can be processed by computing systems?
Usage	Stand-alone → shared	Is the data used only in the project or must be shared across projects or communities? This property is about formats, standards and interoperability
Reproducibility	Store → reproduce	Does the data have to be stored or can it be simply reproduced whenever necessary? The answer depends essentially on the cost and time required to reproduce the data

CPUs could be run on the next generation without too many modifications and with visible improvements in execution speed. Since the advent of multicore and many-core platforms, substantial modifications of existing code and the use of new models of programming, and skills to apply them, are often required in order to obtain performance improvements. Data processing tasks requiring very high performance need often to be optimised to be used on coprocessors, GPUs or emerging combinations of CPUs, GPUs or FPGAs. Further increase in performance of several orders of magnitude is expected to come from new types of architectures designed for specific classes of tasks, like non-von Neumann architectures [8] or quantum processors [9]. Additionally, the use of increasingly bigger caches, fast interconnects, new memory architectures and hardware disaggregation architectures [10] is providing additional performance improvements of the overall computing systems model beyond just the processing units.

3.5.3 Computing Infrastructures

Different types of workloads might have different computing requirements. For example, sequential or parallelisable, but independent, jobs, like BLAST runs, can benefit from a large number of low-core, performance nodes. On the contrary complex simulation jobs with parallelised, but interdependent, jobs can benefit from high-end multicore and many-core CPUs and GPUs. Many scenarios can have both types of requirements for different phases of the workflow. Optimising a data centre for one type of workloads might result in nonoptimal configuration for the other and lack of flexibility in current or future project after the initial infrastructure investments. Setting up facilities able to cope with multiple types of workflows can be expensive and difficult to maintain operational over the facility lifetime.

Commercial procurement of computing resources using the cloud business model is becoming an increasingly affordable way of providing flexibility over relatively long periods of time. In cases where local computing or data facilities already exist or have strategic value, the IaaS model provides the possibility to scale up (more of the same nodes), sideways (different types of nodes) or both depending on projects' requirements while keeping a sound, maintainable baseline infrastructure. Many commercial providers exist today that can provide this type of infrastructure services with many different types of service-level agreements, from widely known companies like Amazon or Microsoft to local service providers reselling resources and adding specialised consultancy and support services.

Much work is being done today on enabling sharing of resources (computing and data) across different cloud infrastructures. Recent releases of the popular OpenStack cloud implementation contain functionality to create federations of cloud across different facilities [11]. However, the issue of providing adapted and flexible governance models, or "governance-as-a-service", for domains of applications where the value of sharing resources strongly depends on the context is still an unresolved issue.

3.5.4 Data Analytics Platforms

Once data has been collected and is safely stored or accessible and computing resources are available or easily procured, the focus can shift to acting on that data and look for valuable insights. Tools and methods to apply models and patterns to datasets have existed for many years, but only recently they have started addressing data analytics over large quantities of data. The high energy physics community has used for years a framework called ROOT providing the "functionalities needed to deal with big data processing, statistical analysis, visualisation and storage" [12]. Statistical computing languages like R are widely used in many different scientific, industrial or financial applications [13]. More recent tools like Hadoop [14] or Spark [15] have been developed with big data analytics in mind and provide features that are optimised for big data storage and offline analysis or near-real-time data streaming, filtering and analysis. They can often be combined together to provide flexible and potentially powerful data analytics systems over a wide range of applications. However, setting up and maintaining such systems is still not trivial.

Many companies today provide specialised services to either design, set up and maintain on-premise data analytics systems or instantiate sophisticated cloud-based scalable platforms, like Cloudera, MapR, Elasticsearch, Microsoft HDInsights or Amazon Elastic MapReduce, to mention just a few.

3.5.5 Machine Learning Platforms

One of the most difficult aspects of data analytics is to come up with models that not only fit the available data nicely but also generalise well to make predictions. As the amount of data increases and the data becomes largely unstructured, finding such models becomes a science on its own.

Ready-to-use machine learning toolboxes have been available since the 1990s when the aspect of solving practical data analytics problems emerged as an additional use of such techniques besides their use in pure AI research. Open-source toolboxes like Shogun [16] become available at the end of the 1990s and are still in active development.

Today practically all the main data analytics platforms come with a machine learning engine of some sort. Mahout [17] was initially designed as a machine learning engine for Hadoop; the Spark project includes the Spark MLlib engine [18]; and Cloudera, one of the founders of Hadoop, provides a machine learning reference implementation called Oryx [19]. Machine learning platforms have been developed by companies like Microsoft, Google or Amazon to power their search engines, business intelligence systems and AI assistants like Cortana or Google Now and are also part of their cloud-based data analytics commercial services. IBM runs a computer system called Watson [20], initially developed as a question-answering machine able to process questions in natural language and since 2012 used in medical decision support systems [21] and other healthcare data analysis applications.

Machine learning has a growing number of applications in many different domains, from general automated pattern recognition and data discovery models to predictive analysis in industrial, financial or commercial applications, process automation, decision support systems and personalisation. A potentially very powerful application is the possibility of generating new unexpected knowledge from data by letting computer systems identify correlations across different scientific domains and suggesting new research directions based on analysis of exceptions or deviations from known patterns. It is worth mentioning that similar concepts are not new. For example, Douglas Hofstadter's and the Fluid Analogies Research Group's work on fluid concepts and creative analogies to teach machines to think goes back to the early 1980s of the last century [22].

3.6   Applications to Healthcare and Biomedical Research

We have described so far a number of service layers or platforms that can be implemented on premise or by using a growing range of commercial and public online services. Although any layer has potential applications in the healthcare and medical research field, typically the layers are built on each other to provide high-level services to domain experts. With this approach in mind, we can explore what are the existing or potential application of data analytics and machine learning platforms in medical research.

Depending on the amount and type of data, computing requirements and objectives, different applications benefit from different architectures and configurations. The following list is a non-exhaustive, but exemplary, classification of a few major application categories:

- *Genomic analysis*: NGS devices can produce increasingly large quantities of data that require new analytics technique to process at scale; storage and transfer of multi-PB datasets can rapidly become a critical bottleneck in research, if not clinical applications. However, the area where genomic data analysis might require advanced analytics and learning techniques is in the integration with other biomedical and behavioural data in the definition of personalised treatments. Access to anonymised genomic databanks can in itself be considered a platform for medical and clinical research or diagnostics support systems.
- *Drug discovery*: assessing the potential effect of drugs on large numbers of possible chemical and biological combinations is a lengthy and costly activity. In silico drug analysis could exploit high-performance computing resources to combine computing simulation with textual description of symptoms and expected outcomes to speed up the identification of compounds and targets and make the process more effective [23].
- *Clinical trials*: analysis of medical records of patients and clinical target data might allow doctors to optimise the design of clinical trials, perform targeted recruitment and enrolment in the different stages of the trials, review and assess pipeline results and therefore increase efficiency and reduce costs.
- *Image analysis*: machine learning-based image content recognition has many applications in medical research or diagnostics; quasi-real-time anatomy localisation or tissue segmentation can become critical in precision medicine, cancer treatment or hybrid surgical rooms where robotics devices can be used to assist the doctors.
- *Clinical decision support systems* (*CDSS*): large-scale data integration and analysis of structured (genomics, EHRs, clinical trial results, etc.) and unstructured information (laboratory notes, doctors' notes, publications, etc.) can become an effective support for personalised diagnostics. Many issues related with sharing personal information and respect of privacy have to be addressed.
- *Trends and simulations*: deep analytics of epidemics data can be used to predict the spread of diseases and better target delivery of cures and optimise logistics and budget; experiments with using not only medical data but data extracted

from social networks and the World Wide Web have been performed in the past few years.

- *Health state definition*: what constitutes healthy behaviour? What prevents it and how to avoid it? This could be the ultimate application of machine learning to healthcare. Collection and analysis of large amounts of personal, medical environmental or behavioural via medical records, wearable devices, social fitness and health platforms could potentially drive the rise of truly personalised healthcare, by preventing rather than curing non-healthy conditions at their root cause. The hype around this subject is matched by the availability of private investments, although so far there is no concrete evidence of the actual possibility of achieving this goal.

Any of the above-described applications could potentially benefit from the availability of public or commercial data analytics and learning platforms. Indeed, a number of such platforms specifically designed for medical research and clinical applications have been and are being set up by many companies, such as IBM, Cerner, Xerox, HCL, Optum and many others. Research projects like MD-Paedigree aim at integrating "biomedical information, data and knowledge for more predictive, individualised, effective and safer paediatric healthcare" [24].

Of particular interest, although still at the level of initial investigations, is the use of consumer-level fitness and health platforms that are emerging with the increasing use of wearable fitness and health monitoring devices. A number of data collection and processing platforms are available today from companies of the like of Microsoft, Apple, Google, Withings or Fitbit. Most of these platforms use machine learning engines to analyse the data and suggest "observations" or "trends"; they produce motivational comparisons within subcommunities of users based on age, gender, level of exercise and other parameters; they suggest "healthy behaviours" by linking, for example, exercise and nutrition information submitted by the users. Although the random and widespread sharing and use of data with third-party entities certainly raise concerns about confidentiality and privacy, the potential for identifying and driving healthy behaviours by applying deep data analytics techniques to large and varied quantities of data should be further assessed.

3.7   International Collaboration and Initiatives

Setting up and operating distributed computing and data analytics platforms for large-scale data-driven applications require considerable resources and expertise that can be put together only through international collaborations. Europe, the USA and other countries worldwide are heavily investing in setting up public cloud computing and data analysis infrastructure for scientific research.

The European Open Science Cloud [25] proposes to create a public, open scientific computing cloud platform by linking public research organisations, eInfrastructures and commercial cloud services to provide trusted, cost-effective services. The ELIXIR [26] initiative is building a distributed infrastructure dedicated to life science and biological data to support research and clinical applications. BioMedBridges [27] is a joint effort of 12 biomedical research infrastructures working on methods and tools to allow data integration for biological, medical, translational and clinical applications. The eTRICKS [28] project funded by the Innovative Medicines Initiative (IMI) and the tranSMART Foundation [29] are addressing the need of common knowledge management and service platforms for data-intensive translational research.

As public data infrastructures and the ongoing efforts to standardise data, formats and methods become more mature and integrated within the researchers' workflows, more advanced public services for data analytics and learning will see the light and possibly realise a vision of truly international, shared, open and cost-effective research in the biomedical field.

Conclusions

Medicine is arguably one of the fields, if not the field, where the most interesting applications of big data will be seen. However, as we hope to have made clear along this chapter, both the IT and the biomedical fields will need to do some housekeeping if we are to see the advancements, promised by many, become real.

The biomedical field should bring some clarity on the map of values that medical data assume in and out of context. It hurts the field to preserve the current conflictive division:

- A research community siding for extreme sharing of clinical data to support repurposing and data mining for novelty discovery, but resisting the invitations to share data that had been purposefully produced for research, by opposing claims of IP protection or even by embracing the discourse of privacy protection
- A clinical community asking for research data sharing, arguing for total transparency of recommendation/safety/claim-backing data, but hindering the sharing of clinical data by mixing arguments of privacy, of potential misinterpretation of decontextualised data, and not the least opposition to administrative interference with practice

It is of utmost importance for the two souls coexisting in the biomedical world, maybe hereby exaggerated for the sake of the narrative, to lay down an agenda aiming at the generation of a conceptualisation, a map, that would allow appropriate dealing with each of the claims and caveats they propose, in a constructive and actionable way.

At the same time, the IT community should accept to take a step back and listen to those requirements expressed by a field that deals with data of social and political value (among others), which have long been tightly regulated (unlike, say, market data or fundamental physics data). This is to produce a reflection on how to exploit and expand the toolkit that already exists, to embrace the need for governance that would often be multiscale.

It is, after all, the same exercise that an individual would legitimately expect from a medical practitioner when upon becoming a patient, he/she would like to think that public health and personalisation-of-care instances have been weighted and negotiated at best for the circumstances, an exercise that, in its imperfection, is repeated several times per day in medicine and in each and every relationship of care and to a different extent in biomedical research as well. Any big data approach and, as an extension, any IT proposition for the biomedical field should accept that not everything has been resolved and should provide tools and services to handle the negotiation of meaning and ultimately the governance that is engraved in the definition itself of the medical field.

IT has made terrific advancements in the last two decades, and big data and the related ML techniques are promising to leap even further away in the next future, hinting at scenarios in which human and machine intelligence will just complement each other, rather than the latter serving the first. This potentially holds the keys to a future of great discoveries in a biomedical field that is waking to an ever-stronger consciousness of the complexity underlying biology and the dynamics of care. But we would like to call for internal and interdisciplinary dialogues to guide progress towards the (not so) utopic scenario we like to envision and away from the dystopic discourse dominating today's conversation.

References

1. Hey T, Tansley S, Tolle K (eds) (2009) The fourth paradigm: data-intensive scientific discovery. Microsoft Research, Cambridge, UK
2. Laney D (2001) 3D data management: controlling data volume, velocity and variety. Gartner, Stamford, CT, USA
3. https://en.wikipedia.org/wiki/Content_delivery_network
4. https://en.wikipedia.org/wiki/Named_data_networking
5. Open Networking Foundation (2010) Software-defined networking: the new norm for networks. https://www.opennetworking.org/images/stories/downloads/sdn-resources/white-papers/wp-sdn-newnorm.pdf
6. Veryard R (1984) Pragmatic data analysis. Blackwell Scientific Publications, Oxford
7. Dean J, Ghemawat S (2004) MapReduce: simplified data processing on large clusters. USENIX: OSDI'04: 6th Symposium on Operating Systems Design and Implementation, San Francisco
8. http://www.micron.com/about/innovations/automata-processing
9. http://plato.stanford.edu/entries/qt-quantcomp/
10. http://research.microsoft.com/en-US/events/wrsc2014/costa14rackscale.pdf
11. https://wiki.openstack.org/wiki/Keystone/Federation/Blueprint
12. https://root.cern.ch/
13. https://www.r-project.org/about.html
14. https://hadoop.apache.org/
15. https://spark.apache.org/
16. http://www.shogun-toolbox.org/
17. http://mahout.apache.org/
18. https://spark.apache.org/mllib/
19. http://oryx.io/

20. http://www.ibm.com/smarterplanet/us/en/ibmwatson/
21. Memorial Sloan-Kettering Cancer Center, IBM to Collaborate in Applying Watson Technology to Help Oncologists (2012) http://www-03.ibm.com/press/us/en/pressrelease/37235.wss
22. Hofstadter D (1995) Fluid concepts and creative analogies: computer models of the fundamental mechanisms of thought. Basic Books, New York, NY, USA
23. Jacq N et al (2008) Grid-enabled virtual screening against malaria. J Grid Comput 6(1):29–43
24. http://www.md-paedigree.eu/about/
25. Jones R (2015) Towards the European science cloud. CERN, Geneva. doi:10.5281/zenodo.16001
26. http://www.elixir-europe.org/
27. http://www.biomedbridges.eu/
28. https://www.etriks.org/
29. http://transmartfoundation.org/

Shared Medical Record, Personal Health Folder and Health and Social Integrated Care in Catalonia: ICT Services for Integrated Care

4

Òscar Solans Fernández, Carlos Gallego Pérez,
Francesc García-Cuyàs, Núria Abdón Giménez,
Manel Berruezo Gallego, Adrià Garcia Font,
Miquel González Quintana, Sara Hernández Corbacho,
and Ester Sarquella Casellas

4.1 Introduction: The Need for a Shared Medical Record of Catalonia (HC3)

The medical record is a dossier of information that arises from contact between the health professional (doctor, nurse, psychologist, physiotherapist, etc.) and the patient and is compiled to ensure the correct care of the patient and their pathologies. It is therefore a valid document from the medical and legal point of view, which contains information of a healthcare, preventive and social nature.

The information compiled and ordered in the medical record constitutes a registry of data essential for the health professionals in the development of their tasks,

Ò. Solans Fernández (✉) • C. Gallego Pérez • F. García-Cuyàs
Fundació TicSalut, Mataró, Barcelona, Spain

Oficina iSalut Department of Health, Government of Catalonia, Catalonia, Spain
e-mail: osolansf@gencat.cat

N. Abdón Giménez • M. Berruezo Gallego • S. Hernández Corbacho
Oficina iSalut Department of Health, Government of Catalonia, Catalonia, Spain

A. Garcia Font
Fundació TicSalut, Mataró, Barcelona, Spain
Department of Health, Government of Catalonia, Catalonia, Spain

M. González Quintana
Department of Health, Government of Catalonia, Catalonia, Spain

E. Sarquella Casellas
Inter-Ministerial Health and Social Care and Interaction Plan, Government of Catalonia, Catalonia, Spain

© Springer International Publishing Switzerland 2017
G. Rinaldi (ed.), *New Perspectives in Medical Records*, TELe-Health,
DOI 10.1007/978-3-319-28661-7_4

both in the medical and healthcare aspects, of attention and curing of the patients, and from other points of view, also fundamental for the health system, such as teaching, research, epidemiological studies, improvement in healthcare quality and the management and administration of the health centres, without forgetting its legal function.

For its very evolution, the medical record faces the challenge of interoperability with the rest of the health system while also having to complete new contents in order to serve as a useful tool for real integral care. In this sense, the contents of the medical records must also advance towards the information related to chronicity and particularly with health and social care. To be able to provide users with true information about the care process offered to them, access should also be allowed to this information in an integrated way. This article includes a brief outline of the challenges and steps being faced in the evolution of the medical record in Catalonia towards a more open setting and with new contents.

Law 41/2002, of 14 November, basic regulator of the autonomy of the patient and of the rights and obligations in terms of medical information and documenta-tion, and its equivalent law in Catalonia (21/2000), establishes "the objective of advancing in the shaping of the sole medical record per patient" and plans for the existence of a system that "facilitates the shared use of medical records between health centres in Catalonia, in order for the patients attended to in diverse centres do not have to undergo repeated examinations and procedures, and that the healthcare services have access to all the medical information available", advising that the "process guarantees the participation of all the agents involved".

Furthermore, the Catalan Health Plan 2011–2015 establishes that the manage-ment of this information, in its entire life cycle, from its compilation to the genera-tion and dissemination of knowledge, is key to the health system and adds that the information management model must consider the following premises:

- The information must be managed in the sphere of the sector, and to do this, a unified model of governance is necessary. This model is the Shared Medical Record of Catalonia (HC3).
- The suppliers must have the commitment to share the information about their patients online.
- The validity and security of the information must be guaranteed.

The Catalan Health System is made up of over 160 different health providers, both in the public and private sectors, which form an integrated healthcare network of public use. The multiplicity of agents in provision has given rise to a majority of these organisations and centres having their own information systems adapted to their specific needs.

This is why in the ICT Strategy of the Department of Health, it was decided to establish a transversal platform of information to be able to share medical informa-tion between health professionals and since 2008 set into motion the Shared Medical Record of Catalonia (HC3) and a year later the Personal Health Folder (Cat @Salut La Meva Salut) in order to empower the citizenry and involve them in the medical

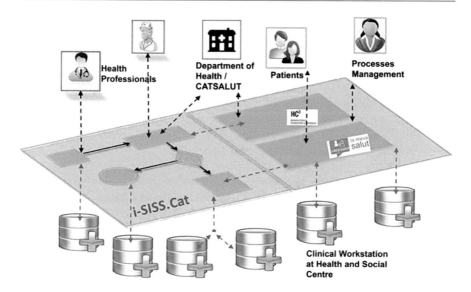

Fig. 4.1 The i-SISS.cat solution

monitoring and in 2014 saw the establishment of the Management System of Integrated Health and Social Care Processes (i-SISS.Cat) which interacts with the different systems of information that make up the current map of medical systems to end up providing support to the derivations and existing healthcare routes between the health and social care providers of Catalonia.

The i-SISS.cat solution will interact with the different information systems that make up the current map of medical systems in Catalonia (Fig. 4.1).

4.2   Fundamental Objectives of the HC3

The HC3 is the electronic model of medical records in Catalonia and encompasses the set of documents that contain data and relevant information about the medical situation and evolution of a patient throughout their healthcare process.

The use of ICT systems, as well as the standards of integration and interoperability that make them compatible, added to the active role of the citizenry, enable having available a sole medical record of the patient focused on health. A common model is thus established of access to registers of the diverse systems of medical information, respecting the differences between providers and entities.

The HC3 is not the sum of the medical records of the different health centres, but a tool that enables the access, in an organised way, to the relevant medical information of the patient, respecting the different models of medical record of the diverse entities.

In the same way, the setting into motion of the HC3 does not mean the elimination of the medical records of the providers, but only a common system of management of the medical information and documentation, specifically its publication and access by the professionals, which must be organised and structured to guarantee the maintenance of an integral model of public use, despite the diversity of models and legal forms of the institutions that provide the services.

Taking into account the variety of entities existent in the Catalan Health System, with different information systems, a model of uniformity is not being imposed but rather of compatibility and interoperability between all of them so that they can share the information, and to achieve this, the characteristics, objectives and basic criteria that the HC3 adopted are the following:

- The main objective is to improve healthcare for the citizenry, by means of an instrument that improves and facilitates the work of the healthcare professionals, on permitting the shared use of the information available between the different healthcare centres.
- Favour the healthcare continuity and contribute to promoting the responsibility of the citizenry towards their own health.
- Improving efficiency, with the decrease of duplicities of tests and with greater control of incompatible treatments, facilitating rationalisation in the use of the resources available.
- Contributing trust in relation to the security and confidentiality of the medical information and accessibility, for both the professionals and the patients.

To achieve these objectives, it is fundamental that the systems of identification of the professionals and of the citizens are completely univocal and that the traceability of all the accesses made to the information is guaranteed.

Nearly 100 % of the centres of the public network are currently connected to the HC3, and in 2015 the rehabilitation and dialysis centres will also be connected. In the coming future, data from the social services and other ambits will be integrated (Fig. 4.2).

The adhesion of the health centres to the HC3 is undertaken through an agreement between them and the Department of Health through which the former promise to comply with the regulation established in the Constitutional Law of Data Protection (LOPD) as well as protecting the data, enabling access only to those authorised professionals and demand from them the appropriate use of the information available.

The agreements to be signed also describe the professional profiles that have access to HC3, as well as the requisites required to do so.

Medical images are also published in the HC3, both radiological and non-radiological. This has been possible due to the project of digitalisation of the images of diagnostic tests that represents a major step forwards in improving healthcare on allowing information to be shared immediately between diverse professionals that have responsibilities in the healthcare process of the patient.

The objectives of this plan are the digitalisation of both radiological and non-radiological medical images. The plan has already achieved, for example, the digitalisation of 100 % of the radiological explorations done in Catalonia, and today we

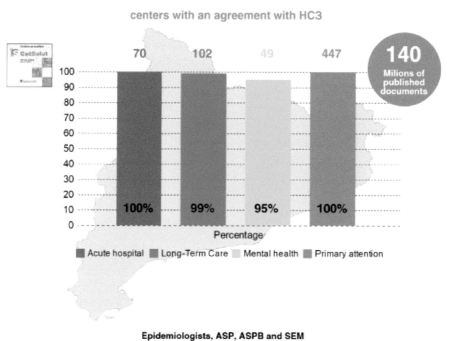

Fig. 4.2 HC3 deployment

are digitalising all the electrocardiograms and structured spirometry tests of primary and specialised healthcare and the non-mydriatic image of the screening of diabetic retinopathy, and we have several of tele-dermatology that is being developed in Catalonia by all the health providers.

4.2.1   HC3 Data of Publication and Access

By means of a series of services and integrations, the health centres publish the most relevant care information of the patients. From the setting into motion of the HC3 to the present, a total of 140 million documents have been published, the publications of the centres growing exponentially. Until August 2015, the publications had increased by 47 % compared to the previous year.

The publications shown in Fig. 4.3 include the global number of publications in HC3 of medical reports, including documents, diagnoses, vaccinations, digital image studies, structured laboratory, spirometry tests and structured pathological anatomy.

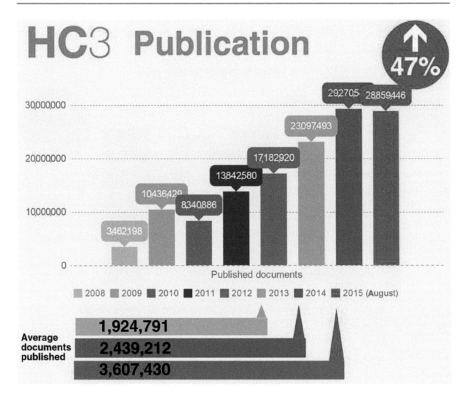

Fig. 4.3 HC3 publication

HC3 gives confidence to the professionals in aspects of security and confidentiality of the data, since it guarantees the traceability of all the accesses and transmission of the information is done securely and univocally.

The professionals can consult the HC3 information in two ways:

- Incorporating the data from HC3 in the medical workstations (ETC) of the centres themselves, all the information in HC3 can currently be integrated into any health information system, always differentiating that the origin of this added information is HC3. Figure 4.4 shows the evolution of the number of applications made to the ETC consultancy service during the last year by month.
- HC3 information can also be consulted by means of the professional visor of the very HC3 system. The professional visor of the HC3 receives a monthly average of 246,401 accesses from professionals. So far this year, this type of access to information has increased by 28 % compared to 2014 (Fig. 4.5).

4.2.2 Technological Basis of HC3

The HC3 is based on the principle of interoperability between the systems. Interoperability is one of the main challenges to overcome in the implementation of information technologies in health. This is confirmed by the majority of actors in

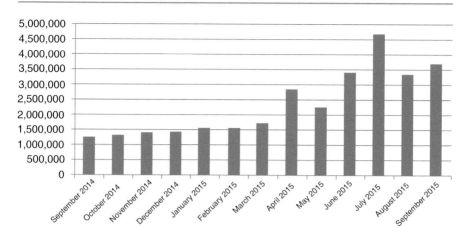

Fig. 4.4 Number of applications made to the ETC

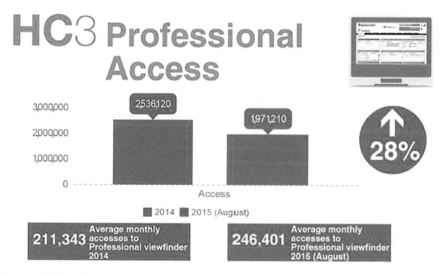

Fig. 4.5 HC3 professional accesses

the system and is reflected in the report developed by Gartner eHealth for a Healthier Europe! Opportunities for a better use of healthcare resources, a study in which the Czech Republic, France, the Netherlands, Sweden, Spain and the United Kingdom have taken part. This report shows that low interoperability between the systems may cause medical errors and increase the frustration of the professional in the use of the medical station.

Interoperability is the capacity that a product or system has, whose interfaces are totally known, to function with other existent or future products or systems and without restriction of access or implementation. We must distinguish between different levels of interoperability (Fig. 4.6).

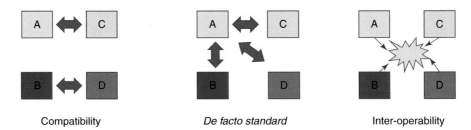

Compatibility   *De facto standard*   Inter-operability

Fig. 4.6 Different levels of interoperability

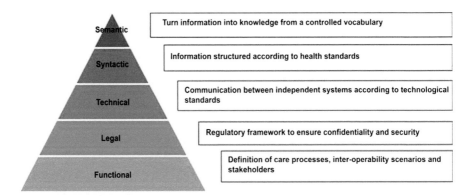

Fig. 4.7 Interoperability process

On the other hand, it is necessary to respond to the need to cover all the healthcare processes of the patient independently of their placement and that of the professionals who attend to them in order to guarantee healthcare continuity.

4.2.3 Interoperability in the Shared Medical Record of Catalonia

Interoperability is a process that can be divided into different levels through which it gradually progresses (Fig. 4.7):

The Shared Medical Record of Catalonia (HC3) has worked and continues working, to achieve the first four levels of interoperability, with the aim of achieving the completion of the semantic level over the next few months in some spheres.

To reach the semantic interoperability, it is necessary to work with international standards that are widely adopted by all the agents, and in health these standards are focused on the syntactic and semantic level.

Below are detailed, for each level of interoperability, the actions that have been undertaken.

4.2.3.1 Functional Interoperability

It is the basis of interoperability. Despite the complexity of the Catalan healthcare model, the Catalan Health System has identified the healthcare processes, the different scenarios of interoperability as well as the most relevant actors that intervene in the exchange of medical information in the HC3.

On the other hand, the diversity of health providers makes it necessary to define a framework of interoperability that enables the guarantee of healthcare continuity.

4.2.3.2 Legal Interoperability

Both Law 21/2000 and the Model Agreement to which the entities from the health system adhere when incorporating into the HC3 cover the legal aspects that permit interoperability between these systems. The guaranteeing aspects of security and confidentiality of the information (use of digital certificates, SAML tokens, application of the data protection law, integration with the auditing system, etc.) are included in this framework.

4.2.3.3 Technical Interoperability

At the end of 2009, the landmark was reached of total incorporation of the SISCAT Catalan Health System centres into the HC3, thus corroborating that the use of standard technologies (SOAP, XML, WS-Security, WSDL, etc.) facilitates communication among the Catalan Health System.

4.2.3.4 Syntactic Interoperability

The HC3 has evolved its formats of information exchange towards structured contents that comply with standard HL7 v3. Gradually, the different entities have adapted their messages to comply with this new standard. For those entities that are in the process of incorporating into the HC3, the messenger service that they must implement to undertake the exchange of information is that which complies with format HL7.

The new functionalities incorporated, such as the results of laboratory tests, pathological anatomy and digital image, have only been defined following standard HL7 v3.

The standard used to share the medical information is the HL7 CDA r2: this standard allows for the progressive incorporation of the structured information.

4.2.3.5 Semantic Interoperability

To achieve interoperability between the systems, it is not enough to achieve the above levels. So that the systems are able to make use of the information exchanged, it is necessary that we use a controlled vocabulary, based on international terminology. For this reason, from HC3, the use of standard semantics is being promoted, as in the case of the use of the benchmark medical terminology SNOMED-CT (in an initial stage, for the pathological anatomy reports) and of LOINC as a standard in the sending of results of laboratory tests (remember that, in both cases, the information is also exchanged in format HL7 CDA r2 level 3). We must also not forget the generalised use of other catalogues of standards such as CIM-9, CIM-10, SERAM or NANDA (Fig. 4.8).

4.2.4 The Current Challenges

The coming challenges of the HC3 in the sphere of interoperability are boosting the exchange of information in HL7 CDA in those systems that at the moment are not

Fig. 4.8 Medical
terminology standards

Information	Format
Pathological anatomy reports	SNOMED-CT
Results of laboratory tests	LOINC
Medical information	CIM-9
	CIM-10
	SERAM
	NANDA

adapted and also to extend the use of SNOMED-CT as a standard of medical terminology in this exchange with the other domains. On the other hand, the effort made
and which is being made to facilitate healthcare continuity at an internal level in
Catalonia enables us to cross the frontiers of the Catalan Health System. The future
is the interconnection at a state level between the systems of the autonomous communities and at a European level through the HCDSNS projects promoted by the
Ministry of Health, Social Services and Equality (MSSSI).

And in the process of continuous improvement with the aim of complying with
Law 49/2007, in reference to equal opportunities, no discrimination and universal
accessibility of disabled persons, the HC3 is committed to accessibility and usability and tools of collaboration, one step further towards human interoperability.

Also the development of new interfaces favours the integration of the HC3 into
the workstations of the professionals, ensuring that the information is not only
accessible through the visor of the professional but also through technical interfaces
(Web services), which enable the health provider to integrate this information into
the information systems under their custody, and ensuring the information reaches
the workstation of the professional. In this way, the care professional has all the
information necessary to take the care decisions, from their workstation, irrespec-
tive of the origin of the information (their own health provider or shared medical
record).

4.2.5   HC3 as ICT Support to the Care Processes to Chronicity

HC3 has accompanied the chronicity strategy in Catalonia with different ICT developments that have made it possible to improve the flows of care of these patients,
giving support to the healthcare route of chronicity between the different health
providers.

HC3 enables the integration of medical data between different centres, the marking of chronic patients, the stratification of risk of the chronic patients showing the
Clinical Risk Group (CRG), the individual intervention plan shared in chronic
patients and the warning system between levels of care to the chronic patient,
between all the different centres of the Catalan public health system.

Fig. 4.9 Total marking
done: (July 2015)

PCC	113,354
MACA	24,837
TOTAL	**138,191**

In 2011 a strategy was initiated of marking complex chronic patients (PCC) and patients with advanced illness (MACA). Since then, all primary health providers have begun to identify these patients (Fig. 4.9).

The different centres of emergencies, hospitals and emergency services such as the 112 telephone integrate this marking into their medical workstations by means of the WS of HC3. Therefore it is an integrated data in the different medical stations and visible in any health centre of the public system.

4.2.6   Shared Individual Intervention Plan (PIIC)

The shared individual intervention plan (PIIC) is a document sustained in the HC3 and which collects the most important health and social data of the patients with complex health needs, placing it in a shared information setting. The proposal is that all PCC or MACA patients have elaborated a PIIC and published in HC3 to be visible in all the centres of the public health system.

It represents an act of communication between professionals, where those that best know a patient synthesise and offer the most relevant information of the case, with the aim that other teams can understand the most essential and thus guarantee that the best decisions are taken in the absence of the professionals of reference, at any time, in any healthcare device.

The PIIC contains information automatically updated about the particulars of the patient, their carers and their professionals of reference, as well as about their health problems, active medication, allergies and results of the multidimensional valuation tests.

Additionally, there are other spheres of information that require that the professional actively introduces them: description of the most probable crisis/imbalances/acuteness and recommendations for their handling, planning of anticipated decisions, information relevant to health and social services that attend to the patient and any other additional information of interest.

The PIIC is drawn up by the professional team in reference to the patient (usually primary care). The patients themselves participate directly in the contents referring to decision-making, so that these are adjusted to their needs and preferences.

Today, more than 100,000 people with complex health needs have PIIC in HC3, and 100 % of health providers can access this information at the moment they attend to the patient.

The preliminary data available inform of the positive impact of the PIIC on the quality and suitability of the 7×24 responses and increase in satisfaction of the patients attended to.

The PIIC project is a singular initiative of the Catalan Health System. Only the Scottish health system is capable of having a similar shared care model.

4.2.7 Evolution and New HC3 Projects: Structured Information

The aim of the HC3 is to have the majority of the information structures, for better operability and monitoring. It began with the laboratory and pathological anatomy which meant a major improvement compared to the initial PDFs:

In the laboratory, the structured information enables comparatives to be made of the patient's results in the professional visor, which facilitates the process of evolution and monitoring.

In pathological anatomy, it facilitates the publication of the results and their integration into the Central Cancer Registry (RCC).

The shared individual intervention plan (PIIC) is a report drawn up in all cases of PCC and MACA markings that has also been structured.

The objective of HC3 is to gradually structure the majority of the information contained in HC3, such as vaccines, diagnoses, allergies or spirometry to facilitate the use and management of it.

Other projects are being developed to improve the HC3 and therefore provide better support to the professionals between the different healthcare levels:

In July 2015 the shared medical course of the patient in HC3 was implemented, the different healthcare centres publishing the objective annotations of medical monitoring in primary healthcare and external consultations of specialised healthcare, with what represents an advance in the improvement of healthcare continuity between the different providers and healthcare levels, avoiding duplicities and increasing security in the healthcare process of each patient.

At the end of 2015, the plan is to incorporate structured medical variables and the incorporation of structured functional scales by all the connected centres.

In brief these evolutions and developments place us in a change of paradigm where the HC3 is no longer a large repository of information but becomes a medical management tool that supports the Catalan Health System.

4.3 Towards the Necessary Exchange of Data Between the Social and Health Integrated Care Systems

Based on the government agreement GOV/28/2014, of 25 February, through which in Catalonia the Interdepartmental Plan of Social and Health Care and Interaction

(PIAISS) was set up, the section of general considerations states "the need to incorporate Information and Communication Technologies (ICT) as an area in which it is considered necessary to establish strategic objectives and guidelines, given the relevance that in collaborative approach of the person and the family it acquires the status of being able to share data between all the healthcare devices involved" and that in the Government Plan 2013–2016 it is made clear that the health and social needs of the population evolve and that the healthcare model must be adapted; strengthen the value of integral healthcare of people and value of the efficiency and quality of the service model, and establish, among its objectives, to promote the combining of social and health services.

In this setting a project is started up to integrate the data between the primary healthcare centres and the social care centres of the different councils using HC3 as an exchange platform.

The Catalan model of integrated care is defined as multidimensional care to people with complex health and social needs. This model is based on the recognition of the active and empowered role of the people attended to as well as in the integral evaluation, the proactive planning and shared practice by the professionals of all the organisations and spheres of care involved. Their objectives are the improvement in the health and well-being results, the adaptation in the use of services and the perception that people have of the care they receive.

In the size of the system, other essential transversal elements must also be guaranteed for the implementation of the model (shared governance, systems of interoperable information, shared vision in the use of resources, framework of common evaluation, models of population stratification and capacitation of the professionals).

In the setting of evolution of the Shared Medical Record and with the aim of increasing the coordination between the social and health services, during 2015, a pilot project has been initiated which analyses how to undertake the integration of the areas of social and health services of the Barcelona City Council. This project includes actions at a functional, technical and legal level.

A model of collaboration of care between health and social services has begun to be built with the intention of sharing data and information of common interest in order to make good medical and care decisions for people with health and social needs.

The idea is to gradually incorporate common goals in the users attended to jointly by the spheres of care and make it easier for the health and social professionals to undertake a valuation process and planning of joint interventions with people who have both health and social needs.

In the context of integrating information from the social services to the HC3, the focus of the solution based on the following premises has been defined:

- The citizenry must authorise the consultation of their social services information by a centre so that the professionals can accede through informed consent that it will be filed in a common repository in HC3 for both systems (Health and Social).

- The citizenry must give its express consent to the access to information of the social services of a centre so that both health and social professionals can access these reports.
- The citizenry must exercise this consent in person at the offices of the council social services or the health centres.
- The HC3 system will provide the communication services to be able to undertake this consent from the applications of the social services centres' systems.
- The advances achieved with the current registry of HC3 and the incorporation of functionalities of the platform should enable the incorporation of a relational space between health and social care, facilitating virtual work and the collaboration between the centres, social workers and other social care professionals. Environments of inter-professional communication must be shaped to encourage this model of collaboration (secure messenger service, etc.).

With all the above, the HC3 system will provide the communication services to be able to make consultations of the data and share it by agreement between the two areas of care (social and health) from the applications of the systems of social services centres.

The healthcare professionals will be able to accede and consult the information authorised by social services of a citizen from the professional visor.

The social services professionals will be able to access specific HCCC information (that which has been agreed between a mixed working commission between professionals from the two spheres) of a citizen through WS in an integrated way in their social workstation.

A Web service is a method of communication between two electronic devices over a network. This will be the way to share information between HCCC (Shared Medical History of Catalonia) and SIAS (Social Service Information System of Barcelona) (Fig. 4.10).

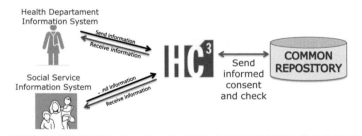

Security	Common repository
→ Informed consent will be signed by the citizen. → The health or social professional will send the document to the common repository . → Each professional can check if the citizen has signed this consent.	→ Informed consent will be custodied in a common repository. → It will be validated by both systems. → It will do periodic checks.

Fig. 4.10 Communication between HC3 and SIAS

HC3 is the first step towards the necessary exchange between the health and social systems in Catalonia. Apart from gradually introducing the improvements and requirements that are made or arise, with the aim of making it more useful to the professionals and friendlier in its use, the future of the HC3 is to transform itself into a real network of information and proactive online services for health and social system professionals as well as the citizenry.

The HC3 is the tool that makes it possible for our health professionals to have access to the relevant medical information about the patient and have a 360° vision of them.

4.4   Personal Health Folder (LMS)

Linked to the HC3, but with its own character, is the Cat@Salut La Meva Salut (Personal Health Folder) project that is based on the right of the citizenry to be able to accede to the information available about their health.

Cat@Salut La Meva Salut (LMS) is a virtual space where the Department of Health makes available to each Catalan citizen the data referring to their health in a secure way, ensuring confidentiality. The aim of the project, however, goes much further than being able to consult medical information, since the goal is for LMS to be an accessible instrument for the citizen, which enables them to interact with their care team and with the health system, to transmit information in all the senses (providing personalised health advice to the citizenry or for them to send the care team the data of regular controls that they do following medical advice), a model that must facilitate the monitoring of pathologies facilitating non-present care (telemedicine and tele-care) whenever this is possible.

LMS has the mission of favouring the self-responsibility of the citizenry regarding their own health, providing them with the information and the tools that enable them to participate in the management of preventative and curative actions, improving the quality of care as well as the coordination between the different lines of services and between the professionals involved.

LMS provides major benefits to the citizenry but also to the providers of services and the administration itself:

It enables the citizen a greater autonomy and comfort in being able to manage processes from their home, such as book appointments, check on pending appointments of any public health centre in an integrated way on the LMS agenda, etc. This year we have started up the econsulta project in Barcelona so that the patient can make a non-present visit to the doctor or nurse from LMS, the professional receiving the visit in an integrated way on their daily agenda and replying from their workstation in a maximum time period of 48 h, all the information being registered in the HIS of the health centre and in LMS. In brief, LMS helps raise awareness among the citizenry to become more responsible for their health since it is a tool focused on monitoring, prevention and monitoring of the medical parameters, being able to become the main source of information about the state of health and which provides them with interaction with the professionals of their health team.

It helps the health providers reduce errors, over-medication and redundancy of tests and other activities, on providing a sole and integrated vision of the medical care that the citizen receives.

It enables the administration to optimise the use of health resources due to the greater commitment of the citizenry regarding their health and the prevention of illnesses, achieving greater efficiency of the system and facilitating the development of all the non-present care.

As regards Web or App services developed or available in health providers of the Catalan Health System, the following criteria of interoperability and standards defined by the Department of Health, LMS, enable any centre to be able to incorporate its apps, being able to undertake personalisation according to the pathologies, needs and interests of each citizen.

With the aim of achieving this interaction in LMS, it is necessary to have a framework of interoperability to ensure that the certified external systems can communicate with LMS, making it essential that they comply with specific specifications relating to communication, portability, identification and publication that have been defined by our Standards Office.

Originally LMS could only be accessed through recognised digital certificates: idCat, eDNI, the National Mint (FNMT), etc. To broaden its use among the population, since 2014, an access system has been in force by means of a robust password. This new system of accreditation for the users of LMS is distributed around all the Primary Healthcare Centres of Catalonia, and since its implementation, the usage data of LMS is increasing more and more.

Suggested Reading

1. http://www.ihtsdo.org/
2. http://www.hl7.org/
3. http://www.msssi.gob.es/profesionales/hcdsns/home.htm

Visual Analytics of Electronic Health Records with a Focus on Time

5

Alexander Rind, Paolo Federico, Theresia Gschwandtner, Wolfgang Aigner, Jakob Doppler, and Markus Wagner

5.1 Introduction

Like many professions, healthcare is facing wide ranging implications rooted in the adoption of information technology. A pivotal healthcare technology is the electronic health record (EHR), which encompasses all health-related data of a patient such as diagnostic parameters, diagnoses, medical history, and past, ongoing, and planned treatments [51]. The availability of these data has great potential to improve decision-making in patient care, quality assurance, and clinical research. Recently, clinical decision support systems embrace methods of machine learning and computational intelligence to semi-automate health choices [34]. However, human inspection and interpretation are still required. For this, EHR systems need to provide physicians, clinicians, and other health professionals with cognitive support in exploring and querying EHRs [10, 51].

This chapter presents visual analytics (VA) as a promising approach to provide healthcare stakeholders such cognitive support in accessing EHRs. After introducing the scientific background of VA, Sect. 5.3 discusses five particular challenges of EHRs and how selected VA projects address them. The chapter closes with an outlook on future research needed.

5.2 Visual Analytics

VA is a young discipline that emerged from the combination of interactive data visualization with concepts from data mining, machine learning, statistics, human

A. Rind (✉) • W. Aigner • J. Doppler • M. Wagner
St. Poelten University of Applied Sciences, St. Poelten, Austria
e-mail: alexander.rind@fhstp.ac.at

P. Federico • T. Gschwandtner
Vienna University of Technology, Vienna, Austria

© Springer International Publishing Switzerland 2017
G. Rinaldi (ed.), *New Perspectives in Medical Records*, TELe-Health,
DOI 10.1007/978-3-319-28661-7_5

computer interaction, and cognitive science [5, 10, 26]. In its research and development agenda ([56], p. 28), VA was defined as

> the science of analytical reasoning facilitated by interactive visual interfaces.

VA has a lot in common with visualization, but its symbiotic approach of combining user interaction with computer-based analysis distinguishes VA from visualization of precomputed analysis results [8]. Thus, we can describe it as

> the method to perform tasks involving data using both computer-based analysis systems and human judgment facilitated by direct interaction with visual representations of data.

In detail this description coins some terms worth discussing (cp. [12, 37]):

Why human judgment?
Computers are nowadays capable to make data-based decisions automatically in a range of scenarios from deleting spam mails to high-frequency trading. It would not make sense to involve humans (or VA) in such time-consuming, repetitive, easy-to-learn, or even distracting tasks, if an existing machine solution is trusted to work sufficiently well.

Still, many scenarios require humans in the loop: Exploratory analysis problems are ill-specified – it is not known in advance what questions will be asked. Background knowledge might be necessary, which cannot all be specified providently in an economic way. VA can also serve as a stepping stone to better understand requirements before developing automatic solutions, to help developers refine automatic solutions, and to determine parameters. Finally, the stakes of a decision might be so high that it cannot be entrusted to a complex black box solution.

Why computer-based analysis systems?
Even though it is possible to visually represent and analyze data by hand, computers enable analysis at a much larger scale: They can update visual representations instantly and thus allow real-time monitoring and interaction. In addition, datasets are often at such scale that they need to be summarized before they can be visually represented. Thus, humans can focus on aspects where their judgment is needed, whereas computers perform steps requiring computational power.

Why visual representations of data?
VA applications display data in the form of a graphic so that visual attributes of the graphic represent data attributes. For example, in a simple bar chart of glucose over time, each bar represents a glucose reading with x-position encoding time and bar length encoding the parameter value. Numbers, text, or tables play only a supportive role in displaying data.

Human cognition can profit from such visual representations in multiple ways: As external memory, they allow to surpass the limitations of human short-term memory capacity. With a suitable spatial layout, the effort to search for items can be reduced, and questions about the data can be answered by perceptual inference, which is easier for humans than reading and comparing values. The human visual system provides a high-bandwidth channel to cognition with extensive preconscious processing in parallel. In contrast to other senses, it is well suited to provide overview of large information spaces.

Why direct interaction and manipulation?
Interaction between human and computer allows the analysts to change their point of view of a dataset, to explore subsets, to highlight connections, etc. VA goes beyond the metaphor of "the human in the loop" and understands the human as steering the analysis loop forward by interaction [15]. Thus, VA applications allow for exploratory analysis in supporting decisions that were unexpected during the applications' development. The pivotal role of interaction is widely acknowledged [1, 42, 55] and illustrated by the VA mantra [27]:

analyse first – show the important – zoom, filter and analyse further – details on demand

Why task- and data-oriented design?
The designers of a VA application need to identify the concrete tasks of a scenario in order to address them effectively. A good solution for one task might be insufficient for another task, even if both tasks involve the same data. Furthermore, this focus on tasks distinguishes VA from visual arts.

In summary, VA is one possible approach for data analysis. Not every scenario can profit from VA – for example, email spam detection involves large numbers of email and is performed sufficiently well by machine learning. Having said that, we think that VA will be particularly useful for the healthcare domain because it features human judgment in a central role and, thus, does not loose background knowledge and empathy. Finally, healthcare decisions are often of a high stake, and an integrated human–machine process as facilitated by VA can gain more trust and meet less resistance than a completely automatic process.

5.3 EHR Challenges for VA

A vibrant research community has emerged on the intersection of VA and healthcare with the VAHC workshop series that is held annually since 2010 in conjunction with either the IEEE VIS conference (e.g., [23]) or the AMIA Annual Symposium (e.g., [11]). In addition, there are dedicated workshops (e.g., [44]) and state-of-the-art reviews (e.g., [51]) on the topic of visualization of EHRs. The rest of this chapter illustrates VA and visualization work with a focus on EHRs. It is structured around technical challenges that were drawn from earlier work [5, 51].

5.3.1 Complexity of Time-Oriented Data

Patients' health status changes over time and, likewise, their prescribed treatment is modified. Encompassing past, present, and future healthcare data, the EHR is a time-oriented dataset. Time has inherent semantic structures comprised of calendar units and contains natural and social cycles like time of day and often irregular reoccurrences like holidays or flu seasons. Therefore, time-oriented data need to be treated differently from other kinds of data and demand appropriate visual representation, interaction, and analytical methods to analyze them.

Surveying visualization of time-oriented data, Aigner et al. [4] identified 13 design aspects. Three aspects have particular implications for EHRs: (i) Time-oriented data can relate to an instant such as the timestamp of a lab test, an interval such as the period of prescription of a drug, or a span such as the minimum time of observation after an operation (see Sect. 5.3.2). (ii) Multiple perspectives of time-oriented data need to be aligned when the EHRs of multiple patients are compared (see Sect. 5.3.3). (iii) Time-oriented data might be given at different levels of temporal precision leading to temporal uncertainty (see Sect. 5.3.4).

5.3.2 Intertwining Patient Condition with Treatment Processes

The data in EHRs is heterogeneous in several aspects. These data may be anchored to instants or intervals of time. LifeLines [43] is a seminal project providing a one-screen overview of an EHR where horizontal lines represent medical problems, hospitalization, or medications, while icons stand for instantaneous events such as doctor consultations, progress notes, or tests.

EHRs contain different data types such as quantitative lab tests, nominal codes for diagnoses and treatment, and frequent passages of free text documentation. VisuExplore [45, 50] provides a selection of chart types for different data types (Fig. 5.1). It was designed with a focus on simple and well-known chart types and extensive interface customization. Quantitative parameters have different units, different measurement methods, and consequently different severity thresholds. The semantic time zoom chart [6, 7] uses color as visual representation of severity in conjunction with an area chart displaying quantitative data. Furthermore, nominal codes found in EHRs can be mapped to a hierarchy such as the ICD-9 classification for diagnoses. An example of using this hierarchy for visual representation of an EHR is the FiveW system [61].

The correct interpretation of both the patient's parameters and the undertaken clinical actions in the context of a specific treatment is a complex analytical task. CareVis [2] presents patient data in combination with computer-interpretable clinical guidelines [41]. CareCruiser [19, 20] extends this approach with a focus on exploring the effects of clinical actions on patient conditions. Since a huge amount of prior domain knowledge is required, Gnaeus [17] utilizes the explicit domain knowledge of guidelines to support the VA process and drive the automated analysis, the visual representation, and the interactive exploration of EHR data (Fig. 5.2).

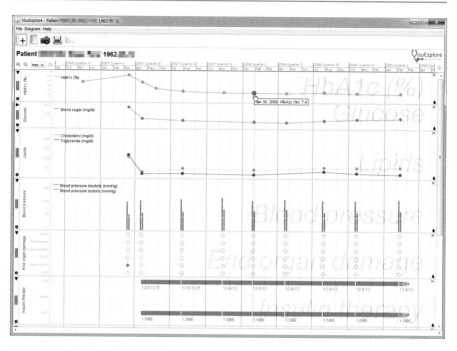

Fig. 5.1 VisuExplore [45, 50]. The screenshot shows an overview of heterogeneous data in the form of diabetes checkup examinations using well-known chart types: *Line plots* for HbA1c, glucose, and lipids; bar chart for blood pressure; event chart for end organ damage; and timeline chart for insulin therapy. The arrangement and the individual views are customizable (With kind permission from Springer Science+Business Media [46])

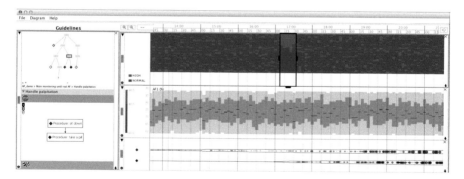

Fig. 5.2 Gnaeus [17], a guideline knowledge-assisted EHR visualization for cohorts, shows the hierarchical (*top left*) and logical (*bottom left*) structure of the clinical guidelines, the temporal abstractions (*top right*), the raw patient data as streaming box plots (*center right*), and the executed clinical actions with their compliance values (*bottom right*) (Image from InfoVis: Wiki.net)

The declarative and the procedural knowledge of the guidelines are exploited to automatically compute temporal abstractions (i.e., clinically meaningful summaries of raw data [54]) and, respectively, compliance values (i.e., the adherence of the actually executed treatments to the guideline recommendations [47]). Temporal abstraction and compliance values then complement and enrich the visualization of raw data; the guideline itself is also visualized, like in CareVis [2] and CareCruiser [19]. Moreover, the guideline knowledge is used to assist the user's interactive exploration of EHR data: when the user navigates the guideline hierarchy and selects a sub-plan, only patient parameters and clinical actions relevant for that sub-plan are visualized.

5.3.3 Scale from Single Patients to Cohorts

Many VA projects do not focus on a single EHR, but aim for insights from analyzing the EHRs of multiple patients in cohorts or even all patients in the EHR system. Possible scenarios are monitoring of patients with chronic diseases, assuring quality of care, and selecting patients for clinical studies or secondary use of EHR data for clinical research.

When multiple EHRs are analyzed together, it is usually more interesting how they develop relative to the start of treatment or another pivotal event in the medical history than to compare them in absolute time. Lifelines2 [58] introduced an interactive control to align event sequences on such pivotal events. CareCruiser [19] and TimeRider [49] are just a few projects demonstrating such interactive alignment.

Space-efficient visual representation techniques make it possible to browse and compare the development of hundreds of EHRs over time. For example, Qualizon Graph [16] combines the space efficiency of Horizon Graph [48] with color-encoded severity levels of semantic time zoom chart [7] to convey a large number of quantitative variables in juxtaposition. LifeFlow [60] focuses on sequences of events such as the arrival at the hospital, transfer to an intensive care unit, or discharge of the patient. EHRs starting with a similar event sequence are aggregated to a tree-based structure and are displayed as colored bars of a height proportional to the number of records in an icicle visualization (Fig. 5.3). The horizontal distance between bars represents the average time between events. More recent work extends this approach for querying sequences of intervals [36], simplification of event data [35], integration of outcomes [59], and comparison of cohorts [32].

When analysts investigate multivariate patterns in EHRs of patient cohorts, they need to visually represent two or more parameters jointly. Gravi++ [25] provides an interactive spring-based layout for multivariate clustering (Fig. 5.4). TimeRider [49] allows bivariate analysis using an animated scatter plot that accounts for data wear by encoding transparency for different sampling rates. MTSA [39] is built as an animated star glyph.

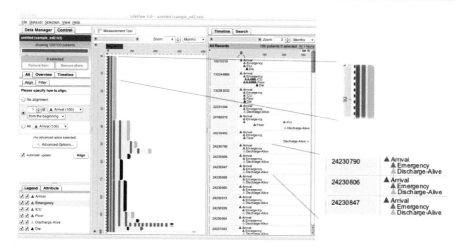

Fig. 5.3 LifeFlow [60] allows exploration of event sequences such as patient transfers between departments. On the right a sequence of three events is displayed in overview and detail (Image from HCIL website reused with permission from C. Plaisant, zoomed details added by the authors)

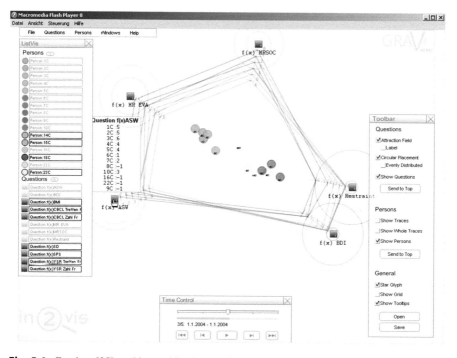

Fig. 5.4 Gravi++ [25] enables multivariate analysis by clustering similar patients in a spring-based layout. Analysts can move the parameter icons (*black squares*) and, thus, influence the layout. Animation and traces allow changes over time to be explored. The screenshot shows additionally the star glyph and rings around parameter icons, which can be used for reading exact values (With kind permission from Springer Science+Business Media [46])

5.3.4 Data Quality and Uncertainty

One important aspect to be considered is the quality of the data. In the medical domain data is often collected via sensors, entered manually by caregivers or patients, or even transcribed from handwritten notes. These types of data collection are prone to data quality problems and may also contain a considerable amount of uncertainty.

One way of handling data quality problems is to build algorithms and visualizations that are tolerant to quality problems and explicitly communicate these problems and uncertainties to the user. Otherwise, these problems could lead to false conclusions about the patient's condition. Another way of dealing with data quality problems is to preprocess the data and to provide interactive means for efficiently identifying and correcting these problems. This process usually requires a human domain expert [28], and thus, VA methods are particularly useful in this matter.

One approach dealing with the problem of data cleansing in the medical domain is described by Lhuillier et al. [31]. They present a set of interactive visualization techniques to help medical practitioners in the digitization and cleansing process of handwritten fluency test results. On the one hand, they provide techniques to support the error-prone process of digitizing the handwritten notes. On the other hand, they provide interactive visualizations to support the identification and correction of implausible entries.

Moreover, special consideration is needed as the characteristics of time-oriented data may induce specific quality problems [21]: for instance, different time scales and precisions of entries, homogeneity of time intervals, entries at impossible times, plausibility of entries at a given point in time, plausibility of entries summing up some values over a given period of time, or plausibility of the sequence of values. Identifying and cleansing such quality problems are the tasks of TimeCleanser [22]. It provides automated as well as visual methods for identifying and correcting suspicious entries (Fig. 5.5). This combination helps to speed up the process, allowing the user to concentrate on quality issues where human judgment is needed.

A related problem is the explicit communication of uncertainty present in the data. There are many approaches to visualize different kinds of uncertainty – some also consider the explicit visualization of temporal uncertainties (e.g., [3, 14, 24, 29]). Besides uncertainty that is inherent in the data (e.g., due to errors of measurement), uncertainty in the data quality or in algorithmic results need to be identified and communicated, in order to enable meaningful reasoning about the data.

5.3.5 User Interaction and User-Centered Design

Section 5.2 emphasized the central role of users in VA and how they can rely on interaction to achieve exploratory tasks. Such tasks are often ad hoc and ill-defined so that the exact sequence of steps taken by users cannot be foreseen

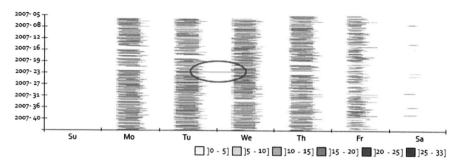

Fig. 5.5 TimeCleanser [22]. The screenshot shows the heatmap view (weekdays are plotted on the x-axis, days are plotted on the y-axis, and the color ranging from *yellow* to *red* indicates the amount of a given value). Besides the general structure of the data, this example shows a few days without entries (maybe holidays) and sporadic entries on Saturdays. Moreover, the visualization reveals one outlier entry at nighttime (*red circle*), which may indicate an error (Image from InfoVis: Wiki.net)

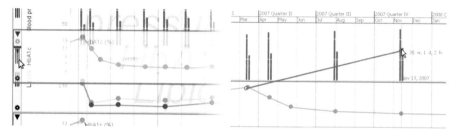

Fig. 5.6 Task-specific interactions in VisuExplore [50]: moving a view (*left*), measurement tape in time (*right*) (With kind permission from Springer Science+Business Media [50])

during application design [52]. Even more so, it is important to rigorously investigate the background and needs of users in a user-centered design process. Ideally, a group of domain experts is available to participate in the design process and for iterative feedback on prototypes. The nested model [37] structures this process in four layers that are recursively nested: domain situation, data/task abstraction, visual encoding/interaction idiom, and algorithm. Each layer builds on the findings from its outer layers and is realized by its inner layers. For example, visual encoding and interaction techniques are designed based on abstracted data and tasks. These techniques are then implemented by an algorithm. A useful structure for investigating a domain situation is the VA design triangle [33] with its corners data–users–tasks.

A suitable level and choice of interaction techniques are essential to the effectiveness of a VA application. The projects presented above feature some excellent examples: overview and detail in LifeFlow [60], brushing and linking in Gravi++ [25], interactive lenses in CareCruiser [19], alignment in Lifelines2 [58], and reconfiguration and time measurement tape in VisuExplore [50] (Fig. 5.6).

It is also worthwhile to experimentally study the effectiveness of interactions: Pohl et al. [46] found some common interaction patterns in log files observed when physicians used either Gravi++ or VisuExplore. Lam [30] studied the costs of interaction and a study of microarray visualization for biologists [53] concluded that consistent interaction techniques were more important for usability than the choice of visual representation techniques.

5.4   Summary and Outlook

This chapter introduced VA as an approach for data analysis that combines the mutual strengths of computer-based analysis and human experts through visual representations of data and direct interaction. This makes it particularly useful for the healthcare domain. Furthermore, the chapters exhibited a selection of state-of-the-art VA projects addressing five technical challenges in analyzing EHRs: (1) The complexity of time-oriented data constitutes a cross-cutting challenge so that all projects need to consider design aspects of time-oriented data in one way or another. (2) As EHRs encompass patient conditions and treatment, they are inherently heterogeneous data. (3) Scaling from single patients to cohorts requires approaches for relative time, space efficiency, and aggregation. (4) Data quality and uncertainty are common issues that need to be considered in real-world projects. (5) A user-centered design process and suitable interaction techniques are another cross-cutting challenge for each and every VA project.

Each of the five discussed challenges implies research gaps to be addressed beyond the work reported in this chapter. Future work is also needed to address the following technical and societal challenges: (6) Domain experts would benefit from making expert knowledge explicit in order to harness it for further analysis and visualization tasks and share it with others [13, 57]. (7) Collaborative analysis requires multiuser systems, which combine multiple devices and screens [9]. (8) In conjunction with EHRs, real-time sensor data can be used – not only from medical devices but also from areas such as ambient-assisted living, sports, wellness, and life logging [18, 38]. (9) Patients take an increasingly active role in managing their own health using so-called personal health records [40].

Acknowledgments We thank Silvia Miksch for valuable inputs and discussions prior to this work. This work was supported by the Austrian Science Fund FWF [grant number P22883].

References

1. Aigner W (2011) Understanding the role and value of interaction: first steps. In: Miksch S, Santucci G (eds) Proceedings of the International Workshop Visual Analytics (EuroVA). Eurographics, Goslar, pp 17–20
2. Aigner W, Miksch S (2006) CareVis: integrated visualization of computerized protocols and temporal patient data. Artif Intell Med 37(3):203–218
3. Aigner W, Miksch S, Thurnher B, Biffl S (2005) PlanningLines: novel glyphs for representing temporal uncertainties and their evaluation. In: Proceedings of the 9th International Conference on Information Visualisation (IV), IEEE, pp 457–463

4. Aigner W, Miksch S, Schumann H, Tominski C (2011) Visualization of time-oriented data. Springer, London
5. Aigner W, Federico P, Gschwandtner T, Miksch S, Rind A (2012) Challenges of time-oriented visual analytics in healthcare. In: Caban JJ, Gotz D (eds) Proceedings of the VisWeek 2012 Workshop on Visual Analytics in Healthcare, pp 17–20
6. Aigner W, Rind A, Hoffmann S (2012) Comparative evaluation of an interactive time-series visualization that combines quantitative data with qualitative abstractions. Comput Graph Forum 31(3):995–1004
7. Bade R, Schlechtweg S, Miksch S (2004) Connecting time-oriented data and information to a coherent interactive visualization. In: Dykstra-Erickson E, Tscheligi M (eds) Proceedings of the ACM SIGCHI Conference on Human Factors in Computing Systems, CHI, pp 105–112
8. Bertini E, Lalanne D (2009) Surveying the complementary role of automatic data analysis and visualization in knowledge discovery. In: Proceedings of the ACM SIGKDD Workshop on Visual Analytics and Knowledge Discovery: Integrating Automated Analysis with Interactive Exploration, VAKD, pp 12–20
9. Blumenstein K,Wagner M, Aigner W (2015) Cross–platform infoVis frameworks for multiple users, screens and devices: requirements and challenges. In: Proceedings of the DEXiS 2015 Workshop on Data Exploration for Interactive Surfaces. Workshop in conjunction with ACM ITS'15, Funchal
10. Caban JJ, Gotz D (2015) Visual analytics in healthcare – opportunities and research challenges. J Am Med Inform Assoc 22(2):260–262
11. Caban JJ, Gotz D, Perer A, Kharrazi H (eds) (2014) Proceedings of the 2014 Workshop on Visual Analytics in Healthcare. Available from: http://www.visualanalyticshealthcare.org/docs/VAHC2014.proceedings.pdf. Cited 6 Nov 2015
12. Card SK, Mackinlay JD, Shneiderman B (eds) (1999) Readings in information visualization: using vision to think. Morgan Kaufmann, San Francisco
13. Chen M, Ebert D, Hagen H, Laramee R, van Liere R, Ma K, Ribarsky W, Scheuermann G, Silver D (2009) Data, information, and knowledge in visualization. IEEE Comput Graph Appl 29(1):12–19
14. Chittaro L, Combi C (2003) Visualizing queries on databases of temporal histories: new metaphors and their evaluation. Data Knowl Eng 44(2):239–264
15. Endert A, Hossain MS, Ramakrishnan N, North C, Fiaux P, Andrews C (2014) The human is the loop: new directions for visual analytics. J Intell Inf Syst 43(3):411–435
16. Federico P, Hoffmann S, Rind A, Aigner W, Miksch S (2014) Qualizon graphs: space-efficient time-series visualization with qualitative abstractions. In: Proceedings of the 2014 International Working Conference on Advanced Visual Interfaces, AVI, ACM, pp 273–280
17. Federico P, Unger J, Amor-Amoros A, Sacchi L, Klimov D, Miksch S (2015) Gnaeus: utilizing clinical guidelines for knowledge-assisted visualisation of EHR cohorts. In: Bertini E, Roberts JC (eds) Proceedings of the EuroVis Workshop on Visual Analytics, EuroVA, Eurographics, pp 79–83
18. Grinter RE, Siek KA, Grimes A (2010) Is wellness informatics a field of human-centered health informatics? Interactions 17(1):76–79
19. Gschwandtner T, Aigner W, Kaiser K, Miksch S, Seyfang A (2011) CareCruiser: exploring and visualizing plans, events, and effects interactively. In: Proceedings of the IEEE Pacific Visualization Symposium (PacificVis), pp 43–50
20. Gschwandtner T, Aigner W, Kaiser K, Miksch S, Seyfang A (2011) Design and evaluation of an interactive visualization of therapy plans and patient data. In: Proceedings of the 25th BCS Conference on Human-Computer Interaction, BCS-HCI, British Computer Society, pp 421–428
21. Gschwandtner T, Gärtner J, Aigner W, Miksch S (2012) A taxonomy of dirty time-oriented data. In: Multidisciplinary research and practice for information systems, Proceedings of the CD-ARES 2012, Springer, Berlin, LNCS 7465, pp 58–72
22. Gschwandtner T, AignerW, Miksch S, Gärtner J, Kriglstein S, Pohl M, Suchy N (2014) Time-cleanser: a visual analytics approach for data cleansing of time-oriented data. In: Lindstaedt S, Granitzer M, Sack H (eds) Proceedings of the 14th International Conference on Knowledge Technologies and Data-driven Business (i-KNOW 2014), ACM, pp 1–8

23. Gschwandtner T, Perer A, Bernard J (eds) (2015) Proceedings of the 2015 Workshop on Visual Analytics in Healthcare. ACM, New York

24. Gschwandtner T, Bögl M, Federico P, Miksch S (2016) Visual encodings of temporal uncertainty: a comparative user study. IEEE Trans Vis Comput Graph 22(1):539–548

25. Hinum K, Miksch S, Aigner W, Ohmann S, Popow C, Pohl M, Rester M (2005) Gravi++: interactive information visualization to explore highly structured temporal data. J Univers Comput Sci 11(11):1792–1805

26. Keim D, Kohlhammer J, Ellis G, Mansmann F (eds) (2010) Mastering the information age – solving problems with visual analytics. Eurographics, Goslar

27. Keim DA, Mansmann F, Schneidewind J, Ziegler H (2006) Challenges in visual data analysis. In: Proceedings of the Tenth International Conference on Information Visualization, IV, pp 9–16

28. Kim W, Choi BJ, Hong EK, Kim SK, Lee D (2003) A taxonomy of dirty data. Data Min Knowl Disc 7(1):81–99

29. Kosara R, Miksch S (2001) Metaphors of movement: a visualization and user interface for time-oriented, skeletal plans. Artif Intell Med 22(2):111–131

30. Lam H (2008) A framework of interaction costs in information visualization. IEEE Trans Vis Comput Graph 14(6):1149–1156

31. Lhuillier A, Hurter C, Jouffrais C, Barbeau E, Amieva H (2015) Visual analytics for the interpretation of fluency tests during Alzheimer evaluation. In: Proceedings of the 2015 Workshop on Visual Analytics in Healthcare, VAHC, ACM, pp 3:1–3:8

32. Malik S, Du F, Monroe M, Onukwugha E, Plaisant C, Shneiderman B (2015) Cohort comparison of event sequences with balanced integration of visual analytics and statistics. In: Proceedings of the 20th International Conference on Intelligent User Interfaces, IUI, ACM, pp 38–49

33. Miksch S, Aigner W (2014) A matter of time: applying a data-users-tasks design triangle to visual analytics of time-oriented data. Comput Graph 38:286–290

34. Moja L, Kwag KH, Lytras T, Bertizzolo L, Brandt L, Pecoraro V, Rigon G, Vaona A, Ruggiero F, Mangia M, Iorio A, Kunnamo I, Bonovas S (2014) Effectiveness of computerized decision support systems linked to electronic health records: a systematic review and meta-analysis. Am J Public Health 104(12):e12–e22

35. Monroe M, Lan R, Lee H, Plaisant C, Shneiderman B (2013) Temporal event sequence simplification. IEEE Trans Vis Comput Graph 19(12):2227–2236

36. Monroe M, Lan R, Morales del Olmo J, Shneiderman B, Plaisant C, Millstein J (2013) The challenges of specifying intervals and absences in temporal queries: A graphical language approach. In: Proceedings of the ACM SIGCHI Conference on Human Factors in Computing Systems, CHI, ACM, pp 2349–2358

37. Munzner T (2014) Visualization analysis and design. AK Peters/CRC, Boca Raton

38. Niederer C, Rind A, Aigner W (2016) Multi-Device Visualisation Design for Climbing Self-Assessment. In: Proceedings of 20th International Conference on Information Visualisation, iV16, IEEE, forthcoming

39. Ordonez P, Oates T, Lombardi ME, Hernandez G, Holmes KW, Fackler J, Lehmann CU (2012) Visualization of multivariate time-series data in a neonatal ICU. IBM J Res Dev 56(5):7–1, 7:12

40. Pagliari C (2015) The changing face of the personal health record: trends and futures in digital empowerment and personalisation. In: Rinaldi G (ed) New perspectives in medical records: meeting the needs of patients and practitioners. Springer (forthcoming)

41. Peleg M (2013) Computer-interpretable clinical guidelines. J Biomed Inform 46(4):744–763

42. Pike WA, Stasko J, Chang R, O'Connell TA (2009) The science of interaction. Inf Vis 8(4):263–274

43. Plaisant C, Mushlin R, Snyder A, Li J, Heller D, Shneiderman B (1998) LifeLines: using visualization to enhance navigation and analysis of patient records. In: Proceedings of the AMIA Symposium, pp 76–80

44. Plaisant C, Miksch S, Gschwandtner T, Malik S (eds) (2014) Proceedings of the IEEE VIS 2014 Workshop on Visualizing Electronic Health Record Data. Available from: http://www.cs.umd.edu/hcil/parisehrvis/. Cited 6 Nov 2015
45. Pohl M, Wiltner S, Rind A, Aigner W, Miksch S, Turic T, Drexler F (2011) Patient development at a glance: an evaluation of a medical data visualization. In: Campos P, Graham N, Jorge J, Nunes N, Palanque P, Winckler M (eds) Proceedings of the IFIP Human-Computer Interaction – INTERACT 2011, Part IV. Springer, Heidelberg, pp 292–299, LNCS 6949
46. Pohl M, Wiltner S, Miksch S, Aigner W, Rind A (2012) Analysing interactivity in information visualisation. KI - Künstliche Intelligenz 26:151–159
47. Quaglini S (2007) Compliance with clinical practice guidelines. Stud Health Technol Inf 139:160–179
48. Reijner H (2008) The development of the horizon graph. In: Bartram L, Stone M, Gromala D (eds) Proceedings of the Vis08 Workshop from Theory to Practice: Design, Vision and Visualization
49. Rind A, Aigner W, Miksch S, Wiltner S, Pohl M, Drexler F, Neubauer B, Suchy N (2011) Visually exploring multivariate trends in patient cohorts using animated scatter plots. In: Robertson MM (ed) EHAWC 2011 and HCII 2011. Springer, Heidelberg, pp 139–148, LNCS 6779
50. Rind A, Aigner W, Miksch S, Wiltner S, Pohl M, Turic T, Drexler F (2011) Visual exploration of time-oriented patient data for chronic diseases: design study and evaluation. In: Holzinger A, Simonic K (eds) USAB 2011. Springer, Heidelberg, pp 301–320, LNCS 7058
51. Rind A, Wang TD, Aigner W, Miksch S, Wongsuphasawat K, Plaisant C, Shneiderman B (2013) Interactive information visualization to explore and query electronic health records. Found Trends Hum Comput Interact 5(3):207–298
52. Rind A, Aigner W, Wagner M, Miksch S, Lammarsch T (2015) Task Cube: a three-dimensional conceptual space of user tasks in visualization design and evaluation. Information Visualization, Published online before print 27 Dec 2015. doi:10.1177/1473871615621602
53. Saraiya P, North C, Duca K (2004) An evaluation of microarray visualization tools for biological insight. In: Proceedings of the IEEE Symposium on Information Visualization, INFOVIS, pp 1–8
54. Shahar Y (1997) A framework for knowledge-based temporal abstraction. Artif Intell 90(1–2):79–133
55. Spence R (2007) Information visualization: design for interaction, 2nd edn. Prentice Hall, Upper Saddle River
56. Thomas JJ, Cook KA (eds) (2005) Illuminating the path: the research and development agenda for visual analytics. IEEE, Los Alamitos, CA, USA
57. Wagner M (2015) Integrating explicit knowledge in the visual analytics process. In: Doctoral Consortium on Computer Vision, Imaging and Computer Graphics Theory and Applications (DCVISIGRAPP 2015), SCITEPRESS Digital Library, Berlin
58. Wang TD, Wongsuphasawat K, Plaisant C, Shneiderman B (2011) Extracting insights from electronic health records: case studies, a visual analytics process model, and design recommendations. J Med Syst 35(5):1135–1152
59. Wongsuphasawat K, Gotz D (2012) Exploring flow, factors, and outcomes of temporal event sequences with the outflow visualization. IEEE Trans Vis Comput Graph 18(12):2659–2668
60. Wongsuphasawat K, Guerra Gomez JA, Plaisant C, Wang TD, Taieb-Maimon M, Shneiderman B (2011) LifeFlow: visualizing an overview of event sequences. In: Proceedings of the ACM SIGCHI Conference on Human Factors in Computing Systems, CHI, pp 1747–1756
61. Zhang Z, Wang B, Ahmed F, Ramakrishnan IV, Zhao R, Viccellio A, Mueller K (2013) The five Ws for information visualization with application to healthcare informatics. IEEE Trans Vis Comput Graph 19(11):1895–1910

Military ICT and Innovative Networks for the Protection of People's Health

6

Giorgio Noera, Tonino Bombardini, Luca Ghetti,
Claudio Camerino, Francesco Frezzetti,
and Antonio Gaddi

6.1 Premise

The European demographic crisis, together with the new socio-economic composition of the population, will lead to a necessary evolution of the healthcare system, which is currently hospital centric.

Demographic shifts and societal changes are intensifying pressures on health systems and demanding new directions in the delivery of healthcare. We are getting older. Ageing populations in both emerging and developed nations are driving up the demand for healthcare.

According to the United Nations, the world's population is expected to increase by one billion people by 2025. Of that billion, 300 million will be people aged 65 or older, as life expectancy around the globe continues to rise. Additional healthcare resources and service innovation is needed globally to deliver the long-term care and chronic disease management services required by a rapidly increasing senior population.

At the same time, developing countries are experiencing significant growth in their middle class. The Brookings Institution estimates 65 % of the global population

Health Ricerca e Sviluppo (HRS) is a public-private organisation that was founded in 2001 as academic spin-off between Alma Mater University of Bologna and Confindustria Emila Romagna (Industrial Trade Union). Presently, HRS is a strategic partner for dual use military and civilian projects within National Plans of Military Research of the Italian Ministry of Defence.
e-mail: presidenza@healthricercaesviluppo.it

G. Noera (✉) • L. Ghetti • C. Camerino • F. Frezzetti • A. Gaddi
Health Ricerca e Sviluppo, Spin off Università di Bologna, Piani Nazionali di Ricerca
Militare a 2012.042 Ministero della Difesa, Bologna, BO, Italy
e-mail: giorgio.noera@gmail.com

T. Bombardini
Istituto di Fisiologia Clinica Consiglio Nazionale delle Ricerche, Pisa, Italy

© Springer International Publishing Switzerland 2017
G. Rinaldi (ed.), *New Perspectives in Medical Records*, TELe-Health,
DOI 10.1007/978-3-319-28661-7_6

will be middle class by 2030. Accelerated urbanisation and access to middle-class comforts are promoting sedentary lifestyle changes that will inevitably lead to greater incidence of obesity, diabetes and other costly health conditions. However, these demographic changes will not be evenly distributed across the globe. For example, growth will be more concentrated in some parts of the world. Africa's population is anticipated to double by 2050, while Europe's population is shrinking old age, when multiple pathologies are common, healing tends to be slower, many treatments are palliative rather than curative and the likelihood of an additional illness or condition arising increases with age.

6.2   Impact on Healthcare

Driven in part by demographic changes, a new paradigm of public and private sector collaboration is developing to transform healthcare financing and delivery. Partnerships with new market participants from industries such as retail, telecommunications, technology, wellness and fitness are expanding and reshaping the health system. What is the payoff for collaborators? These partnerships open the door to a multi-trillion dollar global market for these new commercial entrants, while governments gain access to the innovation and efficiency of new technologies they would not otherwise be able to afford. The shared benefits are long-term cost savings with better outcomes for the patients at a time when changing demographics are depleting health resources.

A rising middle class will fuel increasing demand for more health options. Looking forward, more effective partnerships are needed between the public and private sectors to meet these expectations. Collaborations that in the past may have seemed unlikely will become commonplace. Changing technology and consumer needs will inspire partnership innovations that cut through conventional thinking. As the population grows, technological innovations in mobile health will advance cost-effective health solutions.

Technology and analytics are ushering in new ways of promoting wellness, preventing disease and providing patient-centric care. These advances are exciting tools for providers, private payers and governments alike, as they bring greater precision to predicting patient behaviour and detecting and diagnosing diseases. Different parts of the world will be impacted differently by these demographic shifts. Successful and sustainable change across the globe will require flexible.

6.3   The Objectives

Beyond the current state of art in telehealth and tele-care systems, the aim is to suggest and develop a new approach – using CHC – to develop a civilian integrated healthcare system.

Contributing to the sustainability of the healthcare system may improve clinical decisions based on new diagnostic tools and real-time patient localisation.

Facing the challenges posed by redesigning in- and out-hospital monitoring systems may facilitate the development of integrated care models, with the potential of being more closely oriented to the needs of home-care settings.

6.4   Background

Wireless sensor networks (WSNs) are collection of tiny, low-cost devices with sensing, computing, storing, communication and possibly actuating capabilities. Every sensor node is programmed to interact with the other ones and with its environment, constituting a unique distributed and cooperative system aiming at reaching a global behaviour and result. WSNs are a powerful technology for supporting a lot of different real-world applications, and for a demonstration it is worth noting that in the last decade this new technology has emerged in a wide range of different domains including healthcare, environment and infrastructures monitoring, smart home automation, emergence management and military support, showing a great potential for numerous other applications.

When a WSN is specifically used for being applied to the human body, we deal with wireless body sensor network (WBSN) which involves wireless wearable physiological sensors for strictly medical or non-medical purposes.

For example, they can be very effective for providing continuous monitoring and analysis of physiological or physics parameters very useful, among the others, in medical assistance, in motion and gestures detection, in emotional recognition, etc. Unfortunately, designing such networks is not an easy work because it implies knowledge from many different areas, ranging from low-level aspects of the sensor node hardware and radio communication to high-level concepts concerning final user applications.

Overcoming these difficulties by providing a powerful yet simple software development tool is a fundamental step for better exploiting current sensor platforms. It is quite evident that middleware supporting high-level abstraction model can be adopted for addressing these programming problems and assisting users in a fast and effective development of applications. For this reason, programming abstractions definition is one of the most fermenting research areas in the context of sensor networks, demonstrated by several high-level programming paradigms proposed during the last years.

6.5   Specific Challenge

Designing and programming applications based on WBSN are complex tasks. That is mainly due to the challenge of implementing signal processing intensive algorithms for data interpretation on wireless nodes that are very resource limited and have to meet hard requirements in terms of wearability and battery duration as well as computational and storage resources.

This is challenging because WBSN applications usually require high sensor data sampling rates which endanger real-time data processing and transmission capabilities as computational power and available bandwidth are generally scarce. This is especially critical in signal processing systems, which usually have large amounts of data to process and transmit. WBSN generally rely on a star-based network architecture, which is organised into a coordinator node (PDA, laptop or other) and a set of sensor nodes. The coordinator (often requiring a base station node for the necessary communication capabilities) manages the network; collects, stores and analyses the data received from the sensor nodes; and also can act as a gateway to connect the WBSN with other networks (e.g. the Internet) for remote data access. Sensor nodes measure local physical parameters and send raw or preprocessed data to the coordinator.

The basic functions required by high-level programming tools are to provide standard system services to easily deploy current and future applications and to offer mechanisms for an adaptive and efficient utilisation of system resources. Such tools embrace a wide range of software systems that can be categorised in different classes, each of which characterised by specific features so that, although most WSN applications have common requirements, many different solutions have been proposed in the last years, differing on the basis of the model assumed for providing the high-level programming abstractions. It emerges that none of the proposed application development methodologies can be considered the predominant one. Part of them has peculiar features specifically conceived for particular application domains but lacks in other contexts.

However, among the different programming methodologies, we believe that the exploitation of the agent-oriented programming paradigm to develop WBSN applications could provide the required effectiveness, flexibility and development easiness as demonstrated by the application of agent technology in several other key application domains.

6.6   Signal Processing

Signal processing is needed to extract valuable information from captured data that stems from transient events, such as falls, as well as from trends, such as the onset of fever. WBSN may need to concurrently capture, process and forward information to different stakeholders. Time critical information from both events and trends would go immediately to emergency services, for example, but information that is not sensitive to delays would go to the physician for review later on. It underlines two characteristics of existing embedded technology: Processing data at a given rate consumes less power on average than transmitting the data wirelessly, and reducing the data rate will reduce power consumption for both wireless transceivers and microprocessors.

These characteristics create a trade-off between processing and communication: On-node signal processing will consume power to extract information, but it will also reduce in-network data rate and power consumption. Arbitrary data-rate reduction will lower the transmitted information's fidelity, and for lossy compression schemes, a rate-distortion analysis would need to define the limits of such a reduction.

Therefore, WBSN nodes must break complex signal processing tasks into manageable segments to minimise algorithmic complexity while meeting real-time deadlines. Such efforts will necessitate operating systems that allow access to efficient hardware peripherals. In addition, work is needed to create feature extraction algorithms and classification methods that are effective yet are not so computationally complex that they would be infeasible for resource-constrained hardware. Techniques such as dynamic voltage-frequency scaling or dynamic power management will create opportunities for dynamic adjustment of algorithmic complexity and therefore trade-off energy and fidelity based on an application's predefined or situational needs.

Context awareness and predictive models might better inform and guide processes that control data reduction. Resource constraints challenge WBSN including integer-only math, limited memory (<20 Kb) and limited power consumption, decreases interference among adjacent WBSN and helps maintain privacy. WSNs typically communicate over radioactive radiofrequency (RF) channels between 850 MHz and 2.4 GHz. Unlike WBSN they are challenged by the dramatic attenuation of transmitted signals resulting from body shadowing—the body's line-of-sight absorption of RF energy, which, coupled with movement, causes significant and highly variable path loss.

6.7   Storage

The microelectronics industry is exploring lower power non-volatile memory such as MRAM and RRAM. Consequently, the availability of on-node storage might enhance WBSN functionality. Because long-term data collection often needs no real-time aggregation, on-node storage is a reasonable solution for archiving data, thereby increasing battery life. Longitudinal assessment is insensitive to delay metrics that challenge time-critical monitoring. Some applications might choose to cache data until body channel conditions are more favourable for transmission. Consequently, conditional caching could prolong battery life, decrease form factor or decrease bit errors.

On-node storage could also be used to archive data for signal classification. By storing biokinetic gait patterns over time, for example, a WBSN could learn to classify healthy gait from pathological gait. Such an archive could inform the signal processing routines needed to detect longitudinal trends and instantaneous events (falls).

6.8   Hierarchical Aggregation

WBSN also have a distinctly *hierarchical nature*. They capture large quantities of data continuously and naturalistically, which microprocessors must process to extract actionable information. Data processing must be hierarchical to exploit the *asymmetry of resources*, preserve system efficiency and ensure that data is available when needed.

At the body aggregator, data processing must reveal relationships among body's sensors. With progressively richer resources, more sophisticated and dedicated data mining systems could uncover information related to small and large populations. Each successive hierarchical level must aggregate more data by supporting higher data rates, making more general inferences and archiving more information. Consequently, hardware and software will need to interoperate through multiple levels of infrastructure to share information. Moreover, information gained at each level will provide feedback to and inform the refinement of classification schemes, feature detection algorithms and sensor coordination, placement and design.

Data processing at the sensor node reveals information specific to the sensor's locality. Information, however, might also come from relationships between data collected at multiple sensors over time. The body area aggregator has the important role of combining data from multiple sensors on the body. The aggregator typically possesses a richer collection of resources and a greater energy capacity than the WBSN nodes. In addition to its role as a data fusion centre, the aggregator creates a bridge between the nodes and higher-level infrastructure. It can also offer user interface and can possess its own sensing capabilities.

The convergence of wireless technologies, such as Bluetooth, cellular and IEEE 802.11; interactive user interfaces such as touch screens; and highly capable embedded microprocessors, make newer mobile phones and personal digital assistants attractive hosts for body area aggregation. At the body aggregator, data processing must reveal relationships among a body's sensors.

With progressively richer resources, more sophisticated and dedicated data mining systems could uncover information related to small and large populations. Each successive hierarchical level must aggregate more data by supporting higher data rates, making more general inferences and archiving more information.

Consequently, hardware and software will need to interoperate through multiple levels of infrastructure to share information. Moreover, information gained at each level will provide feedback to and inform the refinement of classification schemes, feature detection algorithms and sensor coordination, placement and design. The convergence of wireless technologies, such as Bluetooth, cellular and IEEE 802.11; interactive user interfaces such as touch screens; and highly capable embedded microprocessors, make newer mobile phones and personal digital assistants attractive hosts for body area aggregation.

6.9   Communication

Communication is essential to node coordination. WBSN are unique in that they attempt to restrict the communication radius to the body's periphery. Limiting transmission range reduces node's workflow area within an Hub and spoke system.

Preserving quality of service (QoS) over traditional wireless links could require one of several approaches, including adaptive channel coding; transmission power scaling; multiple input, multiple output; novel transceiver architecture; and QoS-aware media access protocols. Ultra-wideband communication could help mitigate aspects of this problem in the near future.

Magnetic induction uses magnetic near-field effects to communicate between two coils of wire. Near-field communication typically suffers less path loss than radiative communication, but coil dimensions complicate packaging. Despite this complication, implantable and swallowed sensors have exploited this communication technology.

Body-coupled communication uses the human body as a channel. WBSN transceivers of this nature are either in contact with, or capacitive coupled to, the skin. Body-coupled communication is appealing because little radiated energy is detectable beyond the human body, channels are highly stable, and energy requirements are low.

However, additional research will need to determine the safety of this approach. Future WBSN might implement several types of transceivers to serve situational needs. For example, a sensor node could employ lower data rate, lower power communication transceivers in parallel with higher data rate and higher power transceivers for both longitudinal and critical communication needs. Transceiver diversity could also help mitigate body shadowing.

6.10   Concept Drawing of Military WBSN

The human ancestral adaptive capacity to adverse events resides in the mental and physical response; the thresholds are mutually related with the intensity-time curve.

In critical events (CE), both man made and nature triggered, the efficiency of the response plays a vital role in contrasting and reducing negative impacts on the affected populations. The performance of involved teams plays a key role in the effectiveness of response interventions. The coordination of the operations requires real-time information to deliver effective emergency management. The current order of communications supplies most of what is necessary; however, allowing for a control of individual performances can drastically increase the effectiveness efficiency of the decision maker, especially in under pressure situations.

Unfortunately, designing such networks is not an easy work because it implies knowledge from many different areas, ranging from low-level aspects of the sensor nodes' hardware and radio communication to high-level concepts concerning final user applications.

Overcoming these difficulties by providing a powerful yet simple software development tool is a fundamental step for better exploiting current sensor platforms.

It is quite evident that middleware supporting high-level abstraction model can be adopted for addressing these programming problems and assisting users in a fast and effective development of applications. For this reason, programming abstractions definition is one of the most fermenting research areas in the context of sensor networks, demonstrated by several high-level programming paradigms proposed during the last years.

The development of WBSN for the military represents a sophisticated analysis of biofeedback algorithms, based on frequencies generated by micro-electro-mechanical systems (MEMS) sensors, as well as sensors which provide information on other vital parameters.

Within the recording, it is possible to filter the body harmonics of biodynamic resonance, including those derived from sustained injuries. Multiple vitality and health indicators, including mental status and physical performance, can be recorded and analysed, relying on the related vibrations of the ribcage.

Research and analysis applied to the design of the hardware, together with the inclusion of dry electrodes in the device, allowed for a substantial reduction in the device weight making it easily wearable, also for long durations. The data, as well as the geographic position, are acquired real time and exported in a hybrid architecture of IP radio, local area network and wireless wide area network intercommunication. The overlap between WBSN data and the real-time geographic position was labelled Cyber Health Check (CHC).

Contributing to the sustainability of the healthcare system may improve clinical decisions based on new diagnostic tools and real-time patient localisation.

Facing the challenges posed by redesigning in- and out-hospital monitoring systems may facilitate the development of integrated care models, with the potential of being more closely oriented to the needs of home-care settings.

6.11   The Objectives

Beyond the current state of the art in telehealth and tele-care systems, the aim is to suggest and develop a new approach – using CHC – to develop a civilian integrated healthcare system.

Contributing to the sustainability of the healthcare system may improve clinical decisions based on new diagnostic tools and real-time patient localisation.

Facing the challenges posed by redesigning in- and out-hospital monitoring systems may facilitate the development of integrated care models, with the potential of being more closely oriented to the needs of home-care settings.

6.12   Approach and Methodology

Networking among devices in, on and around the body poses unique challenges for resource allocation, sensor fusion, hierarchical cooperation, QoS, coexistence and privacy.

On the one hand, minimalistic networking techniques increase system runtime and reduce obtrusiveness; on the other hand, sacrificing QoS or privacy is unacceptable for life-critical or sensitive medical applications.

BASNs introduce a wide range of application scenarios, yet it is not certain if a unified network solution is preferable over application-specific protocols and topologies.

Unlike conventional WSNs, WBSN are generally *smaller* (fewer nodes and less area covered) and have *fewer opportunities for redundancy*. Scalability can lead to inefficiencies when working with the two to ten nodes typical of a WBSN. Adding sensor and path redundancy to address node failure and network congestion might not be a viable strategy for a WBSN seeking to minimise form factor and resource usage.

Consequently, the focus must be on generating intelligent and cooperative QoS for the nodes. On-body and in-body (implantable) networks exhibit *heterogeneity* because of placement constraints and sensor requirements.

Wearability requirements can vary drastically across applications.

Some call for multiple wired networks in a single garment; others call for multiple wirelessly networked devices securely attached at various body locations; and still others call for ultraminiature, biocompatible implanted devices with less frequent communication to the outside world.

The large-scale modular customisation of WBSN military into the civilian CHC involves a need for quality function deployment (QFD) methods.

This is defined as a transformation of qualitative user demands into quantitative parameters, so to deploy the quality-forming functions and in order to deploy methods for the achievement of the quality design into subsystems and component parts, and ultimately into specific elements of the manufacturing process. QFD is designed to help planners to focus on characteristics of new or existing products and services from the viewpoints of market segments, company or technology development needs.

QFD helps transforming the customer needs into engineering characteristics and appropriate test methods for a product or service, prioritising the characteristics of each while simultaneously setting development targets for the products and services.

To succeed in developing thriving new products or improve on existing ones is not easy. Studies indicate that as much as somewhere between 35 and 44 % of all products launched are considered failures. It is one thing to actually discover and measure the customers' needs and wants, but, to achieve results, these findings need to be implemented, i.e. translated into company language. Many companies depend on their warranty programmes, customer complaints and inputs from their sales staff to keep them in touch with their customers.

The result is a focus on what is wrong with the existing product or service, with little or no attention on what is right or what the customer really wants. The success of a product or service largely depends on how they meet the customers' needs and expectations. Consequently, more effort is involved in getting the information necessary for determining what the customer truly wants.

This tends to increase the initial planning time in the project definition phase of the development cycle, but it reduces the overall cycle time in bringing a product to the market.

One process-oriented design method constructed to carry out the translation process and make sure that the findings are implemented is quality function deployment (QFD). QFD is a visual connective process that helps teams focus on the needs of the customers throughout the total development cycle. It provides the means for translating customer needs into appropriate technical requirements for each stage of a product/process development life cycle.

It is well documented that the use of QFD can reduce the development time by 50 % and start-up and engineering costs by 30 %. While the structure provided by QFD can be significantly beneficial, it is not a simple tool to use. It is a complex and very time-consuming process to develop the QFD charts.

Among its drawbacks are the complexities of its charts, the vagueness in the data collected and the analysis performed on a rather subjective basis. A review of potential techniques and methods to overcome these problems it was created and introduced in many industrial sectors.

Artificial intelligence techniques such as fuzzy logic and artificial neural networks, together with management and statistical tools such as the Taguchi method, may be proposed to resolve some of QFD's drawbacks.

Then fuzzy logic is reviewed and an introduction to how it can be incorporated within QFD is highlighted. Artificial neural networks are then considered together with what role it can play in helping QFD. As a method to help benchmarking in the house of quality, the Taguchi method is introduced.

Conclusions are then made regarding how to integrate all the techniques and methods together to produce an intelligent systems approach to QFD.

6.13 Fuzzy Logic

Various inputs, in the form of judgements and evaluations, are needed in QFD charts. Normally, the marketing department through questionnaires, interviews and focus groups collects these inputs.

This gives rise to uncertainties when trying to quantify the information. In order to reduce the uncertainty in the data collected, fuzzy logic can be used.

Fuzzy logic can model vagueness in data and/or relationship in a formal way. This technique is able to manipulate fuzzy qualitative data in terms of linguistic variables. This knowledge consists of facts, concepts, theories, procedures and relationships and expressed rules.

6.14 Purpose and Elements Action Tools

Our task will be to transform the WBSN military into a "tracker" and trigger system, with a capacity to assess and report levels of cyber health check awareness, from a health perspective.

In the first stage, the WBSN will be placed within the context of health facilities with interlinkage, integration and legal policies, developed for a CHC programme.

A restricted web platform will be centralised using a clinical report form and online remote monitoring for caregivers. Intensity of care need, mobility of hospital-home care and vice versa, care quality and home-monitoring time will all be integrated within score index maps.

The second stage will involve the audit-based tool that builds on the results of the tracker developed. The diagnostics will assess and report areas of CHC and good practice in order to advice on future actions.

6.15   Expected Impact

Expected results involve reduced hospital admissions and decrease in the days spent within care institutions, improvements in the daily activities, as well as increased quality of life produced by home care through effective use of CHC and better coordination of in- and out-hospital care processes. Additionally, improved cooperation and information exchange among the actors involved in health, social and informal care services are also expected.

The main aims are to demonstrate the effectiveness of agent-based platforms to support programming of WBSN applications and to show how different platforms allow defining the agent behaviour in a real context.

For these purposes a signal processing in-node system specialised for real-time human activity monitoring has been designed and implemented. In particular, the application is able to recognise body postures, movements' e cardiovascular status of assisted livings.

Suggested Reading

1. Vidhyapeeth B (2016). Healthcare analysis via wireless sensor network. IJSRSET 2(2). Print ISSN: 2395-1990. Online ISSN: 2394–4099
2. Sivakumar M, Chitra S, Madhusudhanan B (2016). Wireless sensor network to cyber physical systems: addressing mobility challenges for energy efficient data aggregation using dynamic nodes: sensor letters. American Scientific Publishers 14(8):852–857(6)
3. Hao Y, Foster R (2008). Wireless body sensor networks for health-monitoring applications Published 9 October 2008. Institute of Physics and Engineering in Medicine Physiological Measurement, 29(11)
4. Akyildiz IF et al. (2002). Wireless sensor networks: a survey, Computer Networks 38(4): 393–422

Perspectives in Digital Health and Precision Medicine

7

Francesco Gabbrielli, Giancarmine Russo, Lidia Di Minco, Massimo Casciello, and Gian Franco Gensini

7.1 Digital Health Development: Equilibrium Over Paradox

Innovations in biomedical sciences are frequent, but only a small number can be used in the short term for concrete advantages in patient care. With regard to digital solutions, it usually happens that technological innovations prove to be too complex for practical use after positive evaluations in experimental setting [1], or quite simply, they cannot be applied to real patients who are the ones who should gain most benefit [2, 3].

Such occurrences are often highlighted in risk assessments and cost-benefit studies addressing innovative technologies [4]. Moreover, in healthcare systems the authorization process of digital innovations for clinical practice can generate obstacles as well, since methods and criteria for scientific validation are not well defined [5]. It is of course for understandable ethical reasons that such authorization process cannot be waived and for reasons concerning public resource management as well [6].

Nevertheless, clinical data are analyzed thorough a workflow-based approach which proves to be incompatible with the life cycle of applied digital technologies because of the time required to obtain validated results through the widely used statistical math for biomedical research.

In ICT and robotics, innovation turnover is on average 6 months which means that a technical solution can be considered obsolete just 1 year after its public release.

F. Gabbrielli • G. Russo (✉) • G.F. Gensini
Italian Society for Telemedicine and e-Health, Rome, Italy
e-mail: giancarminerusso@gmail.com

L. Di Minco
New Health Information System, Italian Ministry of Health, Rome, Italy

M. Casciello
Health Information System and Statistics, Italian Ministry of Health, Rome, Italy

© Springer International Publishing Switzerland 2017
G. Rinaldi (ed.), *New Perspectives in Medical Records*, TELe-Health,
DOI 10.1007/978-3-319-28661-7_7

On the other hand, evidence-based medicine (EBM) methods commonly used for drug research are directly carried out in 3-, 5-, or 10-year-long clinical trials that provide the clinical evidences to evaluate digital solutions in healthcare. Moreover, many efforts are necessary to adapt these clinical experiences to the rationale of drug research, and a great deal of time is needed to obtain validated conclusions provided that trials' result is properly conducted [7, 8].

As a consequence, new paradox is arising: technological R&D products cannot be introduced into clinical practice without EBM clinical assessment, but in this way researchers may reach their scientific conclusions when the technology adopted has become outdated and no longer suitable. In other words, the correct application of EBM in digital health produces reliable scientific results; however, by the time these studies are completed, the technology is no longer appliable since it has become obsolete.

Another undesirable effect resulting from the abovementioned issue consists in the long-standing obstacles to organizing effective partnerships with researchers, hi-tech companies, and healthcare managers.

On the other hand, the research inductive approach is still the best way to achieve real progress and discover useful applications. A subjective conclusion may lead to huge mistakes in clinical practice and to unacceptable risks for patients.

In order to have a better understanding of the limitation in the digital health progress caused by the abovementioned paradoxical effect, we can compare the annual number of scientific publications on digital innovations for healthcare in the two most concrete and applied R&D areas: telemedicine and robotic surgery. By collecting data from PubMed-NCBI internet pages (http://www.ncbi.nlm.nih.gov/pubmed), we can observe that there was a significant increase in telemedicine publications since 1992 and in robotic surgery since 1999. Clinical trials in telemedicine and robotic surgery started 1 year later, respectively, in 1993 for telemedicine (4.1 % on a total of 74 publications during that year) and in 2000 for robotic surgery (8.6 % on a total of 81 publications). The rate of telemedicine trials showed a slight increase up to 2005 reaching 9.5 %, and in the following period, the rate further increased and reached 14.7 % in 2014. The rate of robotic surgery trials was stable in a range from 6 to 8 % without any relevant yearly changes (see Tables 7.1 and 7.2).

During the same period, published studies on telemedicine cost and organization effectiveness were growing to a faster rate than clinical trials (see Fig. 7.1). Furthermore, the publication of reviews, effectiveness, and clinical studies had similar trends, maintaining a significant gap compared to the amount of all other publications, which were mainly single-center experience reports which did not collect sufficient data for statistically significant results from an EBM perspective. In Fig. 7.2 a similar situation can be observed also for robotic surgery publications with only two differences: cost analysis studies had more or less the same rate than clinical trials until 2010 and the gap with all other publications in the same field was less significant.

Analysis of 735 "mHealth" publications of PubMed from 2004 shows a statistically significant increasing trend even if the majority of them have been produced after 2012. Fifty-two (7.1 %) clinical trials can be selected within the mHealth

Table 7.1 Telemedicine publications registered on PubMed-NCBI database from 1992 to 2014 and study design percentage rate compared with yearly publications

Years	Total publications	Cost-effectiveness	Organizational effectiveness	Total effectiveness	%	Reviews	%	Clinical trials	%	Other studies	%
1992	47		1	1	2.1	7	14.9		0	39	83.0
1993	74	3	2	5	6.8	5	6.8	3	4.1	61	82.4
1994	123	5	3	8	6.5	9	7.3	1	0.8	105	85.4
1995	355	32	14	46	13.0	53	14.9	4	1.1	252	71.0
1996	458	25	5	30	6.6	48	10.5	11	2.4	369	80.6
1997	659	43	16	59	9.0	71	10.8	21	3.2	508	77.1
1998	789	50	3	53	6.7	81	10.3	24	3.0	631	80.0
1999	812	42	3	45	5.5	105	12.9	29	3.6	633	78.0
2000	825	42	4	46	5.6	136	16.5	31	3.8	612	74.2
2001	725	54	41	95	13.1	107	14.8	37	5.1	486	67.0
2002	722	41	31	72	10.0	110	15.2	46	6.4	494	68.4
2003	767	29	37	66	8.6	124	16.2	52	6.8	525	68.4
2004	816	32	49	81	9.9	146	17.9	63	7.7	526	64.5
2005	814	38	41	79	9.7	135	16.6	75	9.2	525	64.5
2006	870	48	56	104	12.0	113	13.0	83	9.5	570	65.5
2007	887	42	65	107	12.1	130	14.7	99	11.2	551	62.1
2008	1024	48	63	111	10.8	145	14.2	115	11.2	653	63.8
2009	976	48	74	122	12.5	147	15.1	106	10.9	601	61.6
2010	1044	56	83	139	13.3	165	15.8	125	12.0	615	58.9
2011	1224	57	101	158	12.9	222	18.1	121	9.9	723	59.1
2012	1479	67	127	194	13.1	248	16.8	188	12.7	849	57.4
2013	1700	103	175	278	16.4	307	18.1	227	13.4	888	52.2
2014	1643	94	198	292	17.8	318	19.4	242	14.7	791	48.1

Table 7.2 Robotic surgery publications registered on PubMed-NCBI database from 1999 to 2014 and study design percentage rate compared with yearly publications

Years	Total publications	Cost analysis	%	Reviews	%	Clinical trials	%	Other studies	%
1999	52	3	5.8	7	13.5	–	–	56	–
2000	81	9	11.1	9	11.1	7	8.6	58	69.1
2001	83	2	2.4	15	18.1	8	9.6	78	69.9
2002	118	11	9.3	24	20.3	5	4.2	114	66.1
2003	175	11	6.3	40	22.9	10	5.7	128	65.1
2004	231	20	8.7	67	29.0	16	6.9	155	55.4
2005	251	16	6.4	59	23.5	21	8.4	210	61.8
2006	332	26	7.8	76	22.9	20	6.0	226	63.3
2007	412	37	9.0	126	30.6	23	5.6	305	54.9
2008	481	27	5.6	118	24.5	31	6.4	345	63.4
2009	579	41	7.1	150	25.9	43	7.4	368	59.6
2010	636	52	8.2	171	26.9	45	7.1	498	57.9
2011	842	76	9.0	212	25.2	56	6.7	541	59.1
2012	934	92	9.9	235	25.2	66	7.1	597	57.9
2013	1144	118	10.3	334	29.2	95	8.3	772	52.2
2014	1422	142	10.0	402	28.3	106	7.5	56	54.3

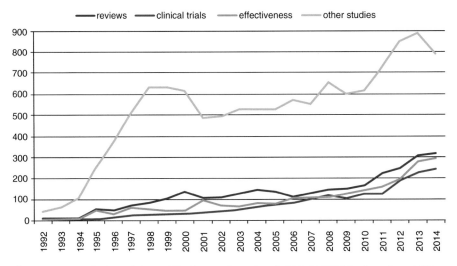

Fig. 7.1 Trend of telemedicine publications registered on PubMed-NCBI database from 1992 to 2014, stratified for study design

group. This new field of investigation is opening the door to other perspectives in digital health, especially with regard to innovative data management strategies and people involvement in data collecting [9–11].

No conclusion concerning the perspectives of digital health can be drawn on the basis of such a simple quantitative analysis of digital health R&D areas, but it is a

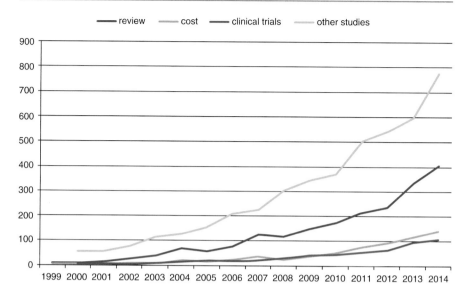

Fig. 7.2 Trend of robotic surgery publications registered on PubMed-NCBI database from 1992 to 2014, stratified for study design

good indicator of the long-standing limits of scientific research on digital innovations for healthcare, and it is also a sufficient basis for the understanding of the persistence of these limits worldwide and in very different economical, social, and organizational environments which cannot of course be considered the cause of the abovementioned issues.

In such situations may happen to register several isolated self-referenced clinical experiences which result in the already well-known negative research fragmentation effects. Current healthcare management decisions are being influenced by them. As a consequence well-known epidemiologic changes due to aging population, increase of chronic diseases, and comorbidities are not managed appropriately.

Thus, strategies for improving the healthcare system have been based just on traditional treatment procedures in conjunction with digital technologies instead of being based on real innovative clinical solutions in digital health. It is noteworthy that different authors in systematic reviews argue that these choices should not be conducted by self-referential theories. In fact, they suggest physicians should take a proactive approach in dealing with the evolution of medical practice in digital health and be aware that the introduction of new technologies in their daily practice is not sufficient to create effective and efficient new digital health services [12–14].

Clinical research methodology [15] and the issues concerning new simulation and experimental validation models [16] for digital health innovations should be brought into question by the scientific international community.

Traditional EBM methods have not yet provided solid scientific validation for digital health clinical studies.

A new approach to evidence-based clinical trials applicable to digital health can be developed, but a coherent healthcare system that provides standard evaluation and projecting criteria methods is needed.

At this time, it appears useful to carry out a detailed evaluation of healthcare cost-efficient measures which are made possible by means of digital health systems. This idea is essentially based on the following widely accepted natural deduction: provided that the realization of one digital health system is necessary to design exact flowcharts on operative procedures, it follows that waste mechanisms will inevitably emerge from the identification of service redundancies or incongruities which can subsequently be removed, thus automatically leading to economic optimization.

Although this line of reasoning is plausible, an overview of international literature shows that there are multiple studies on economic results of digital health which have analyzed a plurality of influencing factors, but the conclusions of these studies have not confirmed the abovementioned idea. In 2001, W.R. Hersh (Oregon Health & Science University, USA) studied the limits in clinical research design with regard to digital services [17].

During the same period of time, at Michigan University (USA) Pamela S. Whitten made an attempt to address the issues pertaining to the economic evaluation of digital health experiences and provide suggestions to solve such issues, by coordinating a systematic review along with other British research groups. Whitten and her collaborators in 2002 published the results of their analysis conducted on 612 experimental studies. Only 55 (9 %) studies have reported data on economic effectiveness, 24 (3.9 %) of them provided cost analysis with validated methods, and none of the studies was eligible for inclusion in meta-analyses [18]. Therefore, a comparison among the abovementioned studies cannot be made, and no conclusions can be drawn on clinical outcomes or economic results.

Furthermore, in 2002, D. Haley published another systematic review on 1300 clinical studies whose outcomes of digital services showed that only 46 (3.5 %) of them reported clinical outcome data suitable for comparison [19].

During the following years, many reviews have highlighted several inconsistencies in the quality of the studies and have attempted to find a way to make possible the comparison of services' outcomes concerning the different technical, medical, and organizational features. Some of them have focused on socioeconomic impacts [20] or standardization assessments [21].

In 2006, W.R. Hersh et al. performed a broad review on 4083 experimental works. From this collection, 597 peer-reviewed and published studies were selected since focused on telemedicine services able to substitute for traditional doctor's appointments. Authors found 97 studies with adequate inclusion criteria for comparative analysis but pointed out that the selected studies did not have a good quality of scientific evidence [22].

The challenges to achieve a validation of a satisfactory level of cost-effectiveness appear to be a consequence of immature technological and organizational levels during the first years of digital health. This is due to the fact that during that period, systematic reviews were focusing on asynchronous digital data generally used in traditional work interactions among health professionals: home telemonitoring for common chronic diseases [23] or emergency teleconsultation [24]. Cost-effectiveness was difficult to demonstrate in emergencies but possible to achieve in chronic disease management, especially if social and familiar costs were evaluated. Nevertheless, the magnitude and significance of telemonitoring of patients' conditions were still deemed inconclusive.

By and large, the same issues have been encountered in recent systematic reviews that have analyzed the period from 2005 to present, in which it is to be noted the substantial maturity of digital technologies and the significant progress made in organizational capability of healthcare systems in the use of digital innovations.

The studies conducted by Victoria Wade et al. (Australia) clearly showed difficulties to compare different digital care settings that were using also better digital health and real-time video communications. The authors screened 3960 clinical experiences and selected 241 articles with economic analyses, and among these, only 36 studies met the inclusion criteria that allowed for the correct assessment of costs and outcomes. Sixty-one percent of telehealth services were found to be less costly than non-telehealth solutions, 31 % of them had greater costs, 3 % had the same costs than non-telehealth services, and in 6 % of telehealth services, the lack of concordance between different analysis perspectives did not allow to reach any conclusion.

Home care services and on-call hospital specialists resulted cost-effective, but the same was not demonstrated when services were provided by interactions between hospital and territorial services for primary care. Finally, the study concluded that the organizational model of care is "more important in determining the value of the service than the clinical discipline, the type of technology, or the date of the study" [25].

By comparing different studies, we can conclude that the analysis of cost-effectiveness has improved over the years, but standardized or at least homogeneous checklists for economic evaluation have not yet been adopted and should be recommended [26].

Current available findings come from several attempts to compare telemonitoring and traditional medical care. This dominant approach limits our present understanding of less common forms of digital services and overall does not facilitate research models neither to compare effectively clinical experiences in different medical or surgical activities [27] nor to consider appropriately patients' adherence to digital services [28] and clinical users' experience evaluation [29], which are key points for a complete economic benefit evaluation.

7.2   From Digital Health to Precision Medicine: Concrete Perspectives

The best and most probable consequence of the progress in ICT is that digital health will make possible a new way to practice medicine. Strengthening prevention and new effective treatments are concrete reasons to dedicate effort and money to realize innovative digital solutions. The criticism toward clinical research methods in digital health we have summarized above adds to the challenge provided by the current limits of biomedical sciences. Thanks to the scientific rationalism, researches have succeeded in providing general rules on several biological and pathological cause-effect mechanisms, and later on, following the results of evidence-based studies, treatments were standardized for different categories of patients. The next step to take is for us to gain insights into interactions of genetic code, metabolism, behavior, and environment that all together describe the personal history of each individual, thus aiming to prevent diseases and be more successful in providing individual therapies. Precision medicine is an emerging medical approach to individual variability. So far it is a little more than a utopian concept on a practical level, but its goals are pivotal if we want to achieve real progress in medicine [30]:

• Improve clinical outcomes and their predictability.
• Reduce the side effects caused by a possibly inappropriate treatment.
• Increase the quality of life.
• Encourage patients' compliance due to a perceived clinical improvement.
• Optimize the use of healthcare resources.

Personalization of treatments in medicine is still a critical issue in most prevalent chronic diseases which are often complicated by comorbidities and also expensive, e.g., asthma [31] or COPD [32]. These conditions require a targeted approach.

Nevertheless, some promising advances have been made and related publications are increasing at a faster rate, such as in the medical PubMed-NCBI database, as shown in Table 7.3.

At this time, the main progresses in precision medicine come more from basic sciences than from clinical trials, but results have been judged interesting enough by the US government to announce on January 20, 2015, the Precision Medicine Initiative® (PMI) that provides for the investment of $215 million to support this initiative in the fiscal year 2016. PMI consists a large-scale cohort of one million or more volunteer US citizens that will allow to gather a large amount of health information and to develop a plan that aims at supporting research activities on cancer genomics of the National Cancer Institute [33].

Firstly, this project collects information from the cohort focused on "way to increase and individual's chances of remaining healthy throughout life" and will

Table 7.3 Precision medicine publications registered on PubMed-NCBI database from 2011 to 2015 (Nov.) and study design percentage rate compared with yearly publications

Years	Total publications	Reviews	%	Clinical trials	%
2011	2	0	–	0	–
2012	21	9		0	–
2013	59	29	49.1	0	–
2014	175	93	53.1	1	0.6
2015	492	113	23.0	5	1.0

also reflect the diversity of the US population with regard to several aspects of their life. The aim is to extend precision medicine to many clinical conditions including common chronic as well as rare illnesses with a new method of engaging research participants, using ICT and integrating different sets of information.

The convergence in one integrated system of digital health with mobile technologies; electronic health records (EHR); data science; genomic, phenotypic, and metabolic analyses; other information sources; and progressive reduction of their costs [34] is the necessary basis for precision medicine development, but a special role in PMI design is played by the innovative methodology that involves the public and is based on their participation in the improvement and maintenance of their own health [35].

One of the most relevant technological progresses pertaining to the genome research discipline is to make ubiquitous core analytical tools once centralized at specialized institutes. In this way, new perspectives have been created, and medical practitioners have been led to use new treatment strategies with their patients. However, healthcare organizations need to increase their capabilities to use "omics" data both in clinical research and in routinary healthcare activities. This implies not only to have adequate tools available (i.e., efficient assembler and aligner, better data interpretation engine) but also to properly address complex datasets used to efficiently support practical decisions, maybe with regard to test order or courses of treatment in one patient as well as comparison of effectiveness of different treatments in different patients.

In literature there are several experiences in accordance with this principle. One of the first evidences is provided by pediatric use of massively parallel sequencing to detect fetal chromosome abnormalities more accurately than the current standard solutions [36]. Genomic programs have also started "encountering many of the same obstacles and developing the same solutions, often independently" in several institutions. Moreover, there are limits on evidences and consensus on the medical significance of genomic variants [37]. This approach needs relevant economic investments and a well-defined pathway to customize healthcare processes [38].

However, advances in human genomics are useful to gain a better understanding of unknown mechanisms which are not anticipated on the basis of phenotype alone, as in the following examples: how the immune system works [39]; the specific antagonism to IL-5 in eosinophilic-driven asthma; identification of patients who will respond to the targeted biological treatment [40]; and identification of one mechanism causing 4 % of cystic fibrosis but effectively treatable [41].

Gaining insights on these mechanisms thanks to genomics seems to be the best way to better understand phenotypic expression [42, 43]. Precision medicine provides the opportunity to interact with other information, thus resulting in a more detailed definition of diagnosis and treatments on the basis of which patients can be stratified for eligibility to different treatments up to individual level. In other words, it will be possible to go initially beyond the traditional treatments toward "phenotype-driven therapy" and to precision or personalized medicine afterwards.

We are not close at achieving these goals yet, but it is urgent to make the first step especially since expensive drugs such as biologics and biosimilars have a negative impact on the sustainability of the healthcare system [44, 45].

References

1. Salisbury C, Thomas C, O'Cathain A, Rogers A, Pope C, Yardley L, Hollinghurst S, Fahey T, Lewis G, Large S, Edwards L, Rowsell A, Segar J, Brownsell S, Montgomery AA (2015) TElehealth in CHronic disease: mixed-methods study to develop the TECH conceptual model for intervention design and evaluation. BMJ Open 5(2):e006448. doi:10.1136/bmjopen-2014-006448
2. Verhoeven F, Tanja-Dijkstra K, Nijland N, Eysenbach G, van Gemert-Pijnen L (2010) Asynchronous and synchronous teleconsultation for diabetes care: a systematic literature review. J Diabetes Sci Technol 4(3):667–684
3. Zanaboni P, Knarvik U, Wootton R (2014) Adoption of routine telemedicine in Norway: the current picture. Glob Health Action 7(22801):1–13. doi:10.3402/gha.v7.22801
4. Frumento E, Colombo C, Borghi G, Masella C, Zanaboni P, Barbier P, Cavoretto D (2009) Assessment and analysis of territorial experiences in digital tele-echocardiography. Ann Ist Super Sanita 45(4):363–371
5. Zanaboni P, Lettieri E (2011) Institutionalizing telemedicine applications: the challenge of legitimizing decision-making. J Med Internet Res 13(3):e72. doi:10.2196/jmir.1669
6. Barlow J, Bayer S, Castleton B, Curry R (2005) Meeting government objectives for telecare in moving from local implementation to mainstream services. J Telemed Telecare 11(Suppl 1): 49–51
7. Whitten P, Holz B, LaPlante C (2010) Telemedicine – what have we learned? Appl Clin Inf 1:132–141, http://dx.doi.org/10.4338/ACI-2009-12-R-0020
8. Fiordelli M, Diviani N, Schulz PJ (2013) Mapping mHealth research: a decade of evolution. J Med Internet Res 15(5):e95. doi:10.2196/jmir.2430
9. Hamine S, Gerth-Guyette E, Faulx D, Green BB, Ginsburg AS (2015) Impact of mHealth chronic disease management on treatment adherence and patient outcomes: a systematic review. J Med Internet Res 17(2):e52. doi:10.2196/jmir.3951
10. Quanbeck AR, Gustafson DH, Marsch LA, McTavish F, Brown RT, Mares ML, Johnson R, Glass JE, Atwood AK, McDowell H (2014) Integrating addiction treatment into primary care using mobile health technology: protocol for an implementation research study. Implement Sci 9:65. doi:10.1186/1748-5908-9-65
11. Bender JL, Yue RY, To MJ, Deacken L, Jadad AR (2013) A lot of action, but not in the right direction: systematic review and content analysis of smartphone applications for the prevention, detection, and management of cancer. J Med Internet Res 15(12):e287. doi:10.2196/jmir.2661
12. Ekeland AG, Bowes A, Flottorp S (2010) Effectiveness of telemedicine: a systematic review of reviews. Int J Med Inform 79:736–771
13. Amadi-Obi A, Gilligan P, Owens N, O'Donnell C (2014) Telemedicine in pre-hospital care: a review of telemedicine applications in the pre-hospital environment. Int J Emerg Med 7:29. doi:10.1186/s12245-014-0029-0, eCollection 2014
14. Zhai YK, Zhu WJ, Cai YL, Sun DX, Zhao J (2014) Clinical- and cost-effectiveness of tele-medicine in type 2 diabetes mellitus: a systematic review and meta-analysis. Medicine (Baltimore) 93(28):e312. doi:10.1097/MD.0000000000000312
15. Wootton R (2012) Twenty years of telemedicine in chronic disease management – an evidence synthesis. J Telemed Telecare 18:211–220. doi:10.1258/jtt.2012.120219
16. Ekeland AG, Bowes A, Flottorp S (2012) Methodologies for assessing telemedicine: a systematic review of reviews. Int J Med Inform 81(1):1–11. doi:10.1016/j.ijmedinf.2011.10.009, Epub 2011 Nov 21
17. Hersh WR, Helfand M, Wallace J, Kraemer D, Patterson P, Shapiro S, Greenlick M (2001) Clinical outcomes resulting from telemedicine interventions: a systematic review. BMC Med Inform Decis Mak 1:5, Epub 2001 Nov 26
18. Whitten PS, Mair FS, Haycox A, May CR, Williams TL, Hellmich S (2002) Systematic review of cost effectiveness studies of telemedicine interventions. BMJ 324:1434–1437
19. Hailey D, Roine R, Ohinmaa A (2002) Systematic review of evidence for the benefits of telemedicine. J Telemed Telecare 8(S1):1–30

20. Jennett PA, Affleck Hall L, Hailey D, Ohinmaa A, Anderson C, Thomas R, Young B, Lorenzetti D, Scott RE (2003) The socio-economic impact of telehealth: a systematic review. J Telemed Telecare 9(6):311–320
21. Demiris G, Tao D (2005) An analysis of the specialized literature in the field of telemedicine. J Telemed Telecare 11(6):316–319
22. Hersh WR, Hickam DH, Severance SM, Dana TL, Krages KP, Helfand M (2006) Telemedicine for the medicare population: update. Evid Rep Technol 131:1–41
23. Paré G, Jaana M, Sicotte C (2007) Systematic review of home telemonitoring for chronic diseases: the evidence base. J Am Med Inform Assoc 14(3):269–277, Epub 2007 Feb 28
24. Brebner JA, Brebner EM, Ruddick-Bracken H (2006) Accident and emergency teleconsultation for primary care – a systematic review of technical feasibility, clinical effectiveness, cost effectiveness and level of local management. J Telemed Telecare 12(Suppl 1):5–8, Review
25. Wade VA, Karnon J, Elshaug AG, Hiller JE (2010) A systematic review of economic analyses of telehealth services using real time video communication. BMC Health Serv Res 10:233. doi:10.1186/1472-6963-10-233
26. Mistry H, Garnvwa H, Oppong R (2014) Critical appraisal of published systematic reviews assessing the cost-effectiveness of telemedicine studies. Telemed J E Health 20(7):609–618. doi:10.1089/tmj.2013.0259, Epub 2014 May 12
27. Kotb A, Cameron C, Hsieh S, Wells G (2015) Comparative effectiveness of different forms of telemedicine for individuals with heart failure (HF): a systematic review and network meta-analysis. PLoS One 10(2):e0118681. doi:10.1371/journal.pone.0118681, eCollection 2015
28. Hameed AS, Sauermann S, Schreier G (2014) The impact of adherence on costs and effectiveness of telemedical patient management in heart failure: a systematic review. Appl Clin Inform 5(3):612–620. doi:10.4338/ACI-2014-04-RA-0037, eCollection 2014
29. Jalil S, Myers T, Atkinson I (2015) A meta-synthesis of behavioral outcomes from telemedicine clinical trials for type 2 diabetes and the Clinical User-Experience Evaluation (CUE). J Med Syst 39(3):28. doi:10.1007/s10916-015-0191-9, Epub 2015 Feb 13
30. Passalacqua G, Canonica GW (2015) AIT (allergen immunotherapy): a model for the "precision medicine". Clin Mol Allergy 13:24. doi:10.1186/s12948-015-0028-6, eCollection 2015
31. Fajt ML, Wenzel SE (2015) Asthma phenotypes and the use of biologic medications in asthma and allergic disease: the next steps toward personalized care. J Allergy Clin Immunol 135(2):299–310. doi:10.1016/j.jaci.2014.12.1871; quiz 311
32. Agusti A (2014) The path to personalised medicine in COPD. Thorax 69(9):857–864. doi:10.1136/thoraxjnl-2014-205507, Epub 2014 Apr 29
33. http://www.nih.gov/precision-medicine-initiative-cohort-program
34. https://www.genome.gov/sequencingcosts/, data from National Human Genome Research Institute (NHGRI)
35. http://www.nih.gov/precision-medicine-initiative-cohort-program/scale-scope
36. Bianchi DW, Parker RL, Wentworth J, Madankumar R, Saffer C, Das AF, Craig JA, Chudova DI, Devers PL, Jones KW, Oliver K, Rava RP, Sehnert AJ, CARE Study Group (2014) DNA sequencing versus standard prenatal aneuploidy screening. N Engl J Med 370(9):799–808. doi:10.1056/NEJMoa1311037
37. Manolio TA, Chisholm RL, Ozenberger B, Roden DM, Williams MS, Wilson R, Bick D, Bottinger EP, Brilliant MH, Eng C, Frazer KA, Korf B, Ledbetter DH, Lupski JR, Marsh C, Mrazek D, Murray MF, O'Donnell PH, Rader DJ, Relling MV, Shuldiner AR, Valle D, Weinshilboum R, Green ED, Ginsburg GS (2013) Implementing genomic medicine in the clinic: the future is here. Genet Med 15(4):258–267. doi:10.1038/gim.2012.157, Epub 2013 Jan 10
38. Hamburg MA, Collins FS (2010) The path to personalized medicine. N Engl J Med 363(4):301–304. doi:10.1056/NEJMp1006304, Epub 2010 Jun 15
39. Zhang Y, Su HC, Lenardo MJ (2015) Genomics is rapidly advancing precision medicine for immunological disorders. Nat Immunol 16(10):1001–1004. doi:10.1038/ni.3275
40. Katz LE, Gleich GJ, Hartley BF, Yancey SW, Ortega HG (2014) Blood eosinophil count is a useful biomarker to identify patients with severe eosinophilic asthma. Ann Am Thorac Soc 11(4):531–536

41. Rowe SM, Heltshe SL, Gonska T, Donaldson SH, Borowitz D, Gelfond D, Sagel SD, Khan U, Mayer-Hamblett N, Van Dalfsen JM, Joseloff E, Ramsey BW, GOAL Investigators of the Cystic Fibrosis Foundation Therapeutics Development Network (2014) Clinical mechanism of the cystic fibrosis transmembrane conductance regulator potentiator ivacaftor in G551D-mediated cystic fibrosis. Am J Respir Crit Care Med 190(2):175–184. doi:10.1164/rccm.201404-0703OC
42. Agache IO (2013) From phenotypes to endotypes to asthma treatment. Curr Opin Allergy Clin Immunol 13(3):249–256. doi:10.1097/ACI.0b013e32836093dd
43. Brasier AR (2013) Identification of innate immune response endotypes in asthma: implications for personalized medicine. Curr Allergy Asthma Rep 13(5):462–468. doi:10.1007/s11882-013-0363-y
44. Bieber T (2013) Stratified medicine: a new challenge for academia, industry, regulators and patients future. Medicine Ltd Unitec House, London. ISBN 978-1-78084-318-6
45. Braido F, Holgate S, Canonica GW (2012) From "blockbusters" to "biosimilars": an opportunity for patients, medical specialists and health care providers. Pulm Pharmacol Ther 25(6):483–486. doi: 10.1016/j.pupt.2012.09.005. Epub 2012 Sep 23; Fuchs VR (2013) The gross domestic product and health care spending. N Engl J Med 369(2):107–109. doi: 10.1056/NEJMp1305298. Epub 2013 May 22.

Medical Record for Clinicians: Present and Future Vision

8

Antonio Vittorino Gaddi

8.1 Medical Record (MR): Prerequisites

Any system of collecting health data must have specific prerequisites. These prerequisites come from ethical, epistemological and logical considerations and from the characteristics of "information" useful to human health; prerequisites cannot be derived only from individual health data analysis or from the needs or requests of clinicians. Figure 8.1 underlines the MR prerequisites (a priori choices in the figure, on the left) deriving from different sources: ethical considerations, identification and syndication of perceived need, agreement of clinicians of "real" needs, technology limits or facilities, research results and others, as discussed in the deep elsewhere [1].

In the literature, several MR characteristics are described (standardisation, semantic interoperability, accessibility, other) [2–7]; however, the a priori choices (mainly ethical, related to patient and citizens' needs) must precede all other technical evaluations, including legal ones.

In other words, there are three steps in the definition of a model for MR construction:

(a) In a first phase, we agree on the general principles (on the left of the figure, which contains only few examples).
(b) Then we decide to define semantic and ontological aspects (central part of the figure).
(c) In a final phase, we build a MR, where technical problems and other details are also taken into account and solved.

A.V. Gaddi
Società Italiana di telemedicina e eHealth, Messina, Italy
e-mail: profgaddi@gmail.com

© Springer International Publishing Switzerland 2017
G. Rinaldi (ed.), *New Perspectives in Medical Records*, TELe-Health,
DOI 10.1007/978-3-319-28661-7_8

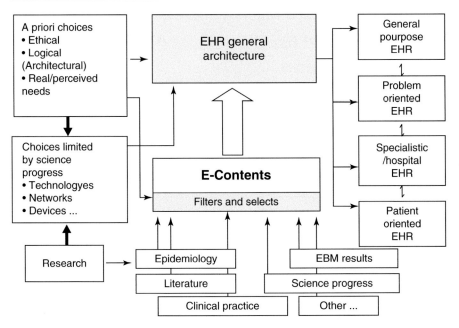

Fig. 8.1 Science-governed and logical approach for the definition of electronic health records (EHR) structure and requirements. The process of producing EHR [1] must start form the *left*. On the *right* some examples of different EHR

So far a converse approach has been used in which the order of the steps is reversed. Sometimes medical records have been created starting from arbitrary choices of some e-contents (ontologies) or using models of strongly disciplinary MR, only suitable for super-specialists. Those are limitations.

Mike Martin, in this book, describes the meaning of the term architecture: "*What Do I need to do before undertaking any technical work*" and proposes the sociotechnical concept of information. That is divided in the socio*cultural view* that takes into account the norms the values and the principals of the information; the *conversional view* that takes into account the role and relationships and the transaction of the information; the *communication view* that takes into account the code and the denotation with who has been transmitted the information; and from the *engineering point of view* that takes into account the amount of information and other technical parameters. This is really a new way for MR architecture in the future.

8.1.1 Prerequisites for Patients, Researchers and Clinicians

However, if the eHealth "*refers to the use of information and communication technologies (ICT) in order to meet the needs of patients, health personnel, citizens and the government*[1,2] then the electronic medical record must contain proper information, useful for this purpose. Such information may be defined as "clinic" as used by doctors to take diagnostic, prognostic and therapeutic decisions. Therefore, the individual information must be accessible by patient/citizen and by other stakeholders of the health process (*"health personnel, government"*). The information must be accessible even in the future, hence must be completed with all the attributes and features and linked with other information, regardless of the current value. In fact, individual data (raw data, coded data, data and knowledge, data collected and coded to lake real – useful – information, etc.) can acquire different values in the future.

This happened several times in the history of medicine.

The electronic medical record is only a part (a relevant part!) of a *wider* system for collection and management of clinical data aimed to *enhance health*.

It is useless, today, that individual institutions or governments propose (or impose) models of electronic medical record. No government, in the past, has proposed medical dossiers "on paper"; therefore, why it has to be done with electronic ones? For example, the Italian *"Fascicolo (= dossier, file) Sanitario elettronico"* is a nationwide model that collects information of an administrative nature and some health documents (pdf). It differs across the country as any regional government (20 in Italy) can modify, change, add components; lacks of the structural basis (architecture); lacks of shared strategic lines, has missing e-contents and semantic tools; lacks of interoperable platforms; does not take in account the need of sharing information among doctors and patients; and the letter in fact has no role at all. This is the wrong way, which perhaps was to be attempted. Nonetheless it remains wrong.

Vice versa, we must collect information *useful to people and doctors. They must be* complete, describing also the context, as defined above.

To define, collect and analyse complex information is a more complex work; however, this work must be done! If we do not, we may find ourselves within a Tower of Babel, with a lot of data without value of information or contradictory, written only on the basis of different medical disciplines, not more manageable, and that can be a source of error. You do not want to take that risk.

An alternative is to not create any architecture at all, with individual scientific institutions and individual physicians creating each time the tools that they need. After a certain number of years (decades) of errors and deaths, secondary to a Darwinian selection, it is likely that a perfect system of eHealth will be born, provided that the "e" still exists in the world. You cannot run a greater risk.

---

[1] Statement of the EU Ministers of Health, Brussels May 22, 2003.

[2] There are other formal definitions of eHealth; a fairly recent is: "eHealth means using digital tools and services for health. eHealth covers the interaction between patients and health-service providers, institution-to-institution transmission of data, or peer-to-peer communication between patients and/or health professionals. Examples include health information networks, electronic health records, telemedicine services, wearable and portable personal health systems and many other information and communication technology (ICT)-based tools assisting disease prevention, diagnosis, treatment and follow up" (EU Action Plan 2010–2020).

In our opinion through adopting a logical, science-driven approach [1] (Fig. 8.1) based on accurate selection of results reported in recent literature, it is possible to create the medical records *functional to scientific research* [8, 9]. This is a fundamental characteristic for the clinical use of electronic medical record (EMR) in the future; cf. below. In fact the EMR should be used both for hospital care and for the home care of the patient [10], which will be, in the near future, the strategic tool for long-life health assurance.[3]

Further relevant topics can be discussed about the requirements of electronic medical records as security, quality certification, privacy, social and legal requirements, standardisation and so on [11–16]; however, in our opinion, all these arguments are not "pre"requisites and have to be discussed when the general architecture of MR has been created.

8.1.2   Focal Point and Priority

We do not need a medical record for the doctors that is equal to or overlaps with the health dossier of people. We do not even need a series of specific clinics folders (ordered for instance by discipline and type of personal health, medical, nursing, etc.) or health dossiers of the patients. What we need to do is to give the possibility to citizens, doctors and researchers to share health information that are useful, complete, updated and linked between them.

Priorities: (a) to create an interoperable platform and a management information system polyvalent, dynamic and universal (not inelastic structures and architectures) and (b) to collect data, we must have *all* data (!) even those of the past, from the patient first and from sites and other sources.

8.2   Electronic Medical Record: No Errors, Please

Electronic medical records might contain and/or cause several errors, ranging from coding errors, errors in prescription of drug or in medicine management in general practice in the diagnostic process up to more complex scenarios [17–21]; they are often related to interaction between pharmacists, physician and patient and may be corrected or prevented by specific methods, as, for example, by "pharmacist-led" information technology-enabled intervention (PRINCE protocol) [19, 21]. Several errors are caused by barriers in retrieving correct clinical data or caused by a failure in data management [22–24] or in conversion of raw data into clinical information. Some errors are trivial (but not for this less serious), as the "copy-and-paste" is wrongly used in electronic medical records [25], or complex and severe, as in the case of the failure to recognise newly identified aortic dilations [26].

---

[3] Crossing point between perceived needs and requirements of the man and the citizen, "requests" for care and capacity of medical/healthcare personnel to "meet the needs" as stated on the definition of eHealth.

Those described up to now are examples of errors and faults in "tactical" management of electronic medical records. However, there are several "strategic" errors, much more serious, related to the general management of the eHealth, including use, misuse or abuse of different medical and personal records and patient summary, the question of the digital divide, the failure data sharing, the difficulties in the formation of the staff, the failure of the empowerment of the citizens [27–34], the inability to overcome the technological barriers [35]. Big faults can be caused by wrong strategic choices, causing "delay and frustration", as reported 10 years after the UK National Health System informatisation [36] with the conclusion that "delivering improved healthcare through nationwide electronic health records will be a long, complex, and iterative process requiring flexibility and local adaptability…." before delivering clinically useful electronic health record systems [36].

For all these considerations, several authors suggested the need of "systemic and continuous" evaluation of all eHealth new projects [37–41].

New criteria for the correct use of clinical information were proposed only recently [9, 10, 42]; therefore, many of the projects of electronic medical records were born too soon, were too much adventurous, or were not designed to fund, not developed enough or did not have sufficient requirements and were not updated.

"Sick patients have more data": so wrote Weiskopf in the title of a recent paper, underlining the relevance of some prototypical definition of EHR completeness: "documentation, breadth, density, and predictive completeness [43]".

What we learn from this literature is not just an analysis of the causes and remedies of such "a great variety of possible errors". This is not the scope of this chapter. What we learn is that "at the beginning", i.e. from the outset, these systems are born already full of pitfalls and errors that might cause damage to the patient or to the citizen. The damage could be found after days, months or years of clinical observation. We need to be conscious of this problem and wondering if there is a case that adopts eHealth criteria (and electronic medical records) similar to those used before drug delivery.

The literature suggests several methods to avoid or control errors. For example, pilot studies before applying to the population the various EMR (and electronic personal record or electronic health dossiers), or to perform a real-time monitoring of the whole population to verify the outcomes, month by month, and not only a few surrogate at the endpoints. The literature also suggests adopting different models of prediction of the risk, for example, FMEA/FMECA (failure mode and effect analysis/failure mode and critical effect analysis) applied to the data retrieved from the electronic health records [23] or to experimental applications of patient summary.[4]

---

[4] Bonora N, Gardellini A, Moretto D, Pettinato A: Failure model & critical Effect Analysis of the Patient Summary NCP38, Val di Setta District, Bologna, Italy. Thesis of the High Course on eHealth of Bologna University (director: Prof AV Gaddi, advisor: Prof F Bonsanto, 2010). *The results of this study have highlighted numerous serious problems and the risk of clinical errors. The results were transmitted to the leaders of regional health. We have no further information.*

8.3   eHealth and Electronic Medical Record: A Disruptive Innovation of Health Systems?

What does disruptive innovation? Disruptive innovation is a concept coined by the US healthcare system and analysed by an "Expert Panel on Effective Ways of Investing in Health" with the idea of analysing ways to improve health outcomes and decreasing health costs, also in the European Union. Disruptive innovation in healthcare is "a type of innovation that creates new networks and new organisational cultures involving new players" with a *potential* improvement of health, displacing "older systems and ways of doing things".

This first assertion, derived from European documents, expresses the utopian idea to do well while spending very little. Maximum yield with minimum expense, as stated by the experts of the trade.

The problem that arises (that has not been discussed enough) is that in the near future many improvements in medicine and the quality (and perhaps amount) of life of patients will depend on the new methods of study of the complexity of the human being. There are, and we hope, heavy investments in research and in clinical research of individuals, in real time, for the study of complex diseases and orphan diseases of drugs, rare or common as they are.

To be able to improve the outcomes by reducing the expenses without knowing the results of this very strong innovation and revolution in medical research is really utopian. It seems more a business and bureaucratic decision that is not guided by science. There is hope ($p = 0.2$) that this may occur *through the eHealth*, If however the instruments used (medical records and all the system of data retrieval, recording, coding, etc.) are designed for this purpose and not hastily to individual needs of disciplinary lobbying (the individual hospitals, the individual scientific societies and so on). The eHealth in fact increases the ability to collect data and to transform it into information; with big data and the advanced computing and with the new models for the analysis of gen-, phen- and environment omics, we can hope for real progress.[5]

It is from a few years that an intense discussion has begun on the disruptive innovation; that takes into account specific medical application (e.g. for the laboratory medicine or for the management of heart in obstetrics and gynaecology) up to possible broad strategic uses [44–49].

The eHealth implementation can fit with the five levels of disruptive innovations (typology of business model, fluency of implementation, health purposes, fields of application and pivoting values) and with five strategic areas (translational research, new innovative technologies, precision medicine, health professional education and health promotion). There are some examples on that direction also for the eHealth application and of telemedicine. More deeply the asynchronous medicine has the

---

[5] Personally, I hope for a holistic revolution that defines a new paradigm to understand the man, of conceptual synthesis and not based (only or mostly) on complicated analysis of large amount of data.

potential to be really disruptive and innovative in respect to our current healthcare processes [50–53].

In the primary care setting, some of the proposals of the expert panel of American College of Physicians [54] open a new innovative and perhaps disruptive way for telemedicine use. In fact: US Physicians support the "expanded role of telemedicine as a method of health care delivery that may enhance patient–physician collaborations, improve health outcomes, increase access to care and members of a patient's health care team, and reduce medical costs when used as a component of a patient's longitudinal care" (first statement of the ACP position paper) [54].

We will have to wait and see. The important thing is that the creation of what today *is only a slogan* (disruptive innovation) to justify economical and political interventions, may be transformed into a true attributes of development, *parallel* to the definition of prerequisites – paragraph 1.0 and reference [55] – and, in general, the structuring of the eHealth (vocals) that is *respectful* of the science and the clinic point of view, particularly in the doctor–patient relationship.

8.4   Final Statement: Systemic or Reductionist Vision?

Premise: you can be pragmatic in both the visions, putting the patient first; the electronic medical record is oriented to cure the patient starting from the first medical encounter or hospital admission. That is called in medicine the "inception point" (basic concept in clinical methodology).

The "need to take care" should not be allowed to choose the pragmatic reductionist vision, let alone to adopt *reductionist* and *simplified tools* (i.e. patient summary or easy-to-use medical records). The medical records are tools for collecting information *useful* to the patient[6]: (a) in the past (rational anamnesis), (b) in the present (= at that precise moment of the life) and (c) in the future, to predict new events (individual prognosis) or health status. Moreover, medical records must also provide that the information should be useful (1) to the patient, (2) to his relative (at present moment) and (3) to offspring (in the present and future), (4) to the patient's community and (5) to clinical research.[7]

Several electronic medical records, at present, are oriented to B1 or AB1 and give priority to the diagnosis, to specialistic treatment and to short-term prognosis.

If data collection systems of the future will be directed only to the specialistic data of a single individual, that will be not possible (it doesn't take anyway). We will never be able to explore the complexity of the man (i.e. of one man) nor create

---

[6] To the patient, to the environment in which he lives, to his wellness, and to the care of his family and other people.

[7] The concept of inception point is essential for the scientific research as to the clinical reasoning on *one individual*, to prognostic aim (P, the main thing), therapy (T, useful to improve the prognosis) and, finally, diagnosis (D, often necessary to formulate P and T; but sometimes used only for taxonomic and disciplinary purposes.

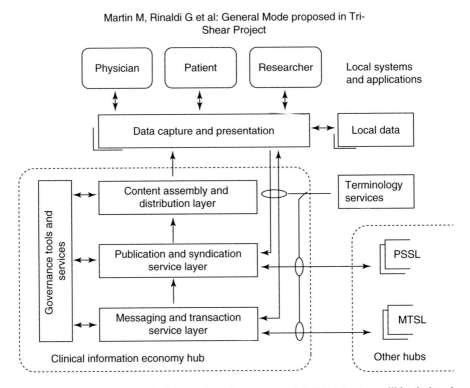

Fig. 8.2 Main components of clinical information economy hub. This structure will be designed at the same time, to the definition of EHR architectures as per Fig. 8.1

science. In this case, the eHealth will serve only to reduce the level of *data-intricacy*, taking advantage of the speed of your computer.

If, vice versa, all the means of telemedicine will contribute to the vision of the system medicine, then perhaps we could explore the *complexity* of the man. This is the main challenge. It is obvious however that this will happen only if the telemedicine tools will have been designed to facilitate this integration and only if the data will be collected (which is neither obvious nor easy). The only alternative is a great deal of confusion.

A rational design of electronic medical record may not be regardless of the creation of a federative interoperable platform. Figure 8.2 shows a general scheme proposed by Martin and Rinaldi et al.[8]

The decision support systems (DSS) to produce a personalised result for individual patients, combining data from genome and biomarkers database and personalised clinical observation, represent one of the innovative tools for the future [56].

Many other innovations are in act or are easily predictable for the foreseeable future. In conclusion, we believe useful to suggest to not activate and do not get to

---

[8] Tri-Shear Project (6th EU Framework Programme, not financed; see Ref. [1] for details).

use our people tools antiquated and not open to future innovation; on the contrary we advise to focus our resources on: (a) the definition, agreed at a supranational level, of templates for the collection of information and (b) on the study of infrastructure tools, capable of solving the semantic and ontological problems and to communicate between people doctors and researchers.

References

1. Rinaldi G, Capello F, Gaddi AV (2013) Medical data, information economy and federative networks: the concepts underlying the comprehensive electronic clinical record framework. Nova Science Publication, New York
2. Martinez-Costa C, Kalra D, Schulz S (2014) Improving EHR semantic interoperability: future vision and challenges. Stud Health Technol Inform 205:589–593
3. Tao C, Jiang G, Oniki TA, Freimuth RR, Zhu Q, Sharma D et al (2013) A semantic-web oriented representation of the clinical element model for secondary use of electronic health records data. J Am Med Inform Assoc: JAMIA 20(3):554–562, Pubmed Central PMCID: 3628064
4. Marcos M, Maldonado JA, Martinez-Salvador B, Bosca D, Robles M (2013) Interoperability of clinical decision-support systems and electronic health records using archetypes: a case study in clinical trial eligibility. J Biomed Inform 15:2–9
5. Avillach P, Coloma PM, Gini R, Schuemie M, Mougin F, Dufour JC et al (2013) Harmonization process for the identification of medical events in eight European healthcare databases: the experience from the EU-ADR project. J Am Med Inform Assoc JAMIA 20(1):184–192, Pubmed Central PMCID: 3555316
6. Hsu W, Taira RK, El-Saden S, Kangarloo H, Bui AA (2012) Context-based electronic health record: toward patient specific healthcare. IEEE Trans Inform Technol Biomed Publ IEEE Eng Med Biol Soc 16(2):228–234
7. Gomoi VS, Dragu D, Stoicu-Tivadar V (2012) Virtual medical record implementation for enhancing clinical decision support. Stud Health Technol Inform 180:118–122
8. Weiskopf NG, Hripcsak G, Swaminathan S, Weng C (2013) Defining and measuring completeness of electronic health records for secondary use. J Biomed Inform 15:2–9
9. Weiskopf NG, Weng C (2013) Methods and dimensions of electronic health record data quality assessment: enabling reuse for clinical research. J Am Med Inform Assoc: JAMIA 20(1):144–151, Pubmed Central PMCID: 3555312
10. Weir CR, Staggers N, Gibson B, Doing-Harris K, Barrus R, Dunlea R (2015) A qualitative evaluation of the crucial attributes of contextual information necessary in EHR design to support patient-centered medical home care. BMC Med Inform Decis Making 15:30, Pubmed Central PMCID: 4416274
11. Farzandipour M, Sadoughi F, Ahmadi M, Karimi I (2010) Security requirements and solutions in electronic health records: lessons learned from a comparative study. J Med Syst 34(4):629–642
12. Zimlich R (2015) Pilot program will explore giving patient access to Ehr records. Med Econ I92(6):59
13. Hoerbst A, Schabetsberger T, Hackl W, Ammenwerth E (2009) Requirements regarding quality certification of electronic health records. Stud Health Technol Inform 150:384–388
14. Lloyd D, Kalra D (2003) EHR requirements. Stud Health Technol Inform 96:231–237
15. Kluge EH (2003) Security and privacy of EHR systems – ethical, social and legal requirements. Stud Health Technol Inform 96:121–127
16. Kalra D, Tapuria A, Austin T, De Moor G (2012) Quality requirements for EHR archetypes. Stud Health Technol Inform 180:48–52
17. Enos N, Enos M (2013) Three EHR-related coding errors to avoid. MGMA Connexion Med Group Manag Assoc 13(5):59

18. Cresswell KM, Sadler S, Rodgers S, Avery A, Cantrill J, Murray SA et al (2012) An embedded longitudinal multi-faceted qualitative evaluation of a complex cluster randomized controlled trial aiming to reduce clinically important errors in medicines management in general practice. Trials 13:78, Pubmed Central PMCID: 3503703
19. Avery AJ, Rodgers S, Cantrill JA, Armstrong S, Cresswell K, Eden M et al (2012) A pharmacist-led information technology intervention for medication errors (PINCER): a multicentre, cluster randomised, controlled trial and cost-effectiveness analysis. Lancet 379(9823):1310–1319
20. Friesner DL, Scott DM, Rathke AM, Peterson CD, Anderson HC (2011) Do remote community telepharmacies have higher medication error rates than traditional community pharmacies? Evidence from the North Dakota Telepharmacy Project. J Am Pharmacists Assoc JAPhA 51(5):580–590
21. Avery AJ, Rodgers S, Cantrill JA, Armstrong S, Elliott R, Howard R et al (2009) Protocol for the PINCER trial: a cluster randomised trial comparing the effectiveness of a pharmacist-led IT-based intervention with simple feedback in reducing rates of clinically important errors in medicines management in general practices. Trials 10:28, Pubmed Central PMCID: 2685134
22. Pantazos K, Lauesen S, Lippert S (2011) De-identifying an EHR database – anonymity, correctness and readability of the medical record. Stud Health Technol Inform 169:862–866
23. Edinger T, Cohen AM, Bedrick S, Ambert K, Hersh W (2012) Barriers to retrieving patient information from electronic health record data: failure analysis from the TREC Medical Records Track. AMIA Annu Symp Proc AMIA Symp AMIA Symp 2012:180–188, Pubmed Central PMCID: 3540501
24. Keenan G, Yakel E, Dunn Lopez K, Tschannen D, Ford YB (2013) Challenges to nurses' efforts of retrieving, documenting, and communicating patient care information. J Am Med Inform Assoc: JAMIA 20(2):245–251, Pubmed Central PMCID: 3638178
25. Brown J (2014) Be wary of copy-and-paste EHR mistakes. Behav Healthcare 34(6):29–30
26. Gordon JR, Wahls T, Carlos RC, Pipinos II, Rosenthal GE, Cram P (2009) Failure to recognize newly identified aortic dilations in a health care system with an advanced electronic medical record. Ann Intern Med 151(1):21–27, W5
27. Kim EH, Kim Y (2010) Digital divide: use of electronic personal health record by different population groups. Conference proceedings: annual international conference of the IEEE engineering in medicine and biology society IEEE engineering in medicine and biology society conference. 2010:1759–1762
28. Kim EH, Stolyar A, Lober WB, Herbaugh AL, Shinstrom SE, Zierler BK, et al (2007) Usage patterns of a personal health record by elderly and disabled users. AMIA Annual Symposium proceedings/AMIA Symposium AMIA Symposium. 409–413. Pubmed Central PMCID: 2655817
29. Yamin CK, Emani S, Williams DH, Lipsitz SR, Karson AS, Wald JS et al (2011) The digital divide in adoption and use of a personal health record. Arch Intern Med 171(6):568–574
30. Rudd P, Frei T (2011) How personal is the personal health record?: comment on "the digital divide in adoption and use of a personal health record". Arch Intern Med 171(6):575–576
31. Tierney WM, Rotich JK, Smith FE, Bii J, Einterz RM, Hannan TJ (2002) Crossing the "digital divide:" implementing an electronic medical record system in a rural Kenyan health center to support clinical care and research. Proceedings/AMIA Annual Symposium AMIA Symposium.792–795. Pubmed Central PMCID: 2244335
32. Quantin C, Benzenine E, Auverlot B, Jaquet-Chiffelle DO, Coatrieux G, Allaert FA (2011) Empowerment of patients over their personal health record implies sharing responsibility with the physician. Stud Health Technol Inform 165:68–73
33. Ammenwerth E, Schnell-Inderst P, Hoerbst A (2011) Patient empowerment by electronic health records: first results of a systematic review on the benefit of patient portals. Stud Health Technol Inform 165:63–67
34. Munir S, Boaden R (2001) Patient empowerment and the electronic health record. Stud Health Technol Inform 84(Pt 1):663–665
35. Shah MN, Morris D, Jones CM, Gillespie SM, Nelson DL, McConnochie KM et al (2013) A qualitative evaluation of a telemedicine-enhanced emergency care program for older adults. J Am Geriatr Soc 61(4):571–576

36. Robertson A, Cresswell K, Takian A, Petrakaki D, Crowe S, Cornford T et al (2010) Implementation and adoption of nationwide electronic health records in secondary care in England: qualitative analysis of interim results from a prospective national evaluation. BMJ 341:c4564, Pubmed Central PMCID: 2933355
37. Catwell L, Sheikh A (2009) Evaluating eHealth interventions: the need for continuous systemic evaluation. PLoS Med 6(8):e1000126, Pubmed Central PMCID: 2719100
38. Sheikh A, Cornford T, Barber N, Avery A, Takian A, Lichtner V et al (2011) Implementation and adoption of nationwide electronic health records in secondary care in England: final qualitative results from prospective national evaluation in "early adopter" hospitals. BMJ 343:d6054, Pubmed Central PMCID: 3195310
39. Segall N, Saville JG, L'Engle P, Carlson B, Wright MC, Schulman K et al (2011) Usability evaluation of a personal health record. AMIA Annu Symp Proc AMIA Symp AMIA Symp 2011:1233–1242, Pubmed Central PMCID: 3243224
40. Hayrinen K, Lammintakanen J, Saranto K (2010) Evaluation of electronic nursing documentation – nursing process model and standardized terminologies as keys to visible and transparent nursing. Int J Med Inform 79(8):554–564
41. Sanderson H, Adams T, Budden M, Hoare C (2004) Lessons from the central Hampshire electronic health record pilot project: evaluation of the electronic health record for supporting patient care and secondary analysis. BMJ 328(7444):875–878, Pubmed Central PMCID: 387482
42. Weiskopf NG, Hripcsak G, Swaminathan S, Weng C (2013) Defining and measuring completeness of electronic health records for secondary use. J Biomed Inform 46(5):830–836, Pubmed Central PMCID: 3810243
43. Weiskopf NG, Rusanov A, Weng C (2013) Sick patients have more data: the non-random completeness of electronic health records. AMIA Annu Symp Proc AMIA Symp AMIA Symp 2013:1472–1477, Pubmed Central PMCID: 3900159
44. Stein D, Chen C, Ackerly DC (2015) Disruptive innovation in academic medical centers: balancing accountable and academic care. Acad Med: J Assoc Am Med Coll 90(5):594–598
45. Shaikh AT, Ferland L, Hood-Cree R, Shaffer L, McNabb SJ (2015) Disruptive innovation can prevent the next pandemic. Front Publ Health 3:215, Pubmed Central PMCID: 4585064
46. Rifai N, Topol E, Chan E, Lo YM, Wittwer CT (2015) Disruptive innovation in laboratory medicine. Clin Chem 61(9):1129–1132
47. Felker GM, Ahmad T (2015) Reclassifying heart failure: time for disruptive innovation? Eur J Heart Fail 17(9):879–880
48. Gee RE (2014) Disruptive innovation in obstetrics and gynecology: the Robert Wood Johnson Clinical Scholars Program (1972–2017). Curr Opin Obstet Gynecol 26(6):493–494
49. Eckert SE (2014) Does disruptive innovation enhance our paradigm shifts? Int J Oral Maxillofac Implants 29(4):771–772
50. Grady J (2014) CE: Telehealth: a case study in disruptive innovation. Am J Nurs 114(4):38–45, test 6–7
51. Reiner BI (2013) Commoditization of PACS and the opportunity for disruptive innovation. J Digit Imaging 26(2):143–146, Pubmed Central PMCID: 3597945
52. Yellowlees PM, Odor A, Parish MB (2012) Cross-lingual asynchronous telepsychiatry: disruptive innovation? Psychiatr Serv 63(9):945
53. Yellowlees P, Odor A, Patrice K, Parish MB, Nafiz N, Iosif AM et al (2011) Disruptive innovation: the future of healthcare? Telemed J e-health: Off J Am Telemed Assoc 17(3):231–234
54. Daniel H, Sulmasy LS, Health ACP, Public Policy C (2015) Policy recommendations to guide the use of telemedicine in primary care settings: an American College of Physicians Position Paper. Ann Int Med 194–199
55. Gaddi AV, Manca M, Capello F (2013) eHealth, care and quality of life. Springer, Milan
56. Kouris I, Tsirmpas C, Mougiakakou SG, Iliopoulou D, Koutsouris D (2010) E-Health towards ecumenical framework for personalized medicine via Decision Support System. Conference proceedings: Annual International Conference of the IEEE Engineering in Medicine and Biology Society IEEE Engineering in Medicine and Biology Society Conference. 2010:2881–2885

Addressing eHealth at the EU Level

9

Terje Peetso

9.1 Electronic Health Records: What EU Does?

The important role of eHealth in health and social care systems has been widely recognised in the EU Member States. The European Commission is supporting them in
implementing eHealth in their healthcare systems through different activities including the work towards the deployment of electronic health records (EHR), for which
considerable investments have been made for decades. In the 1990s the work focused
mainly on the development of EHR and connectivity within a point of care or maximum within a health delivery system at local/regional/national level. Although these
objectives have not yet been fully achieved, the work is now aiming at creating possibilities for having an access to health information across borders. However, the main
goal has remained the same – to enable fast access to vital information and sharing of
information among health professionals to improve access to quality and efficiency of
care. Several documents and EU-wide projects support reaching this goal:

- The Commission Communication 'Europe 2020: A strategy for smart, sustainable and inclusive growth' underlines the importance of eHealth by stressing the
  need to promote deployment and usage of modern accessible online services
  including eHealth [1].
- The Digital Agenda Europe [2] strategy addressed eHealth capability to support
  independent living for ageing citizens, revolutionise health services and deliver
  better public services at a lower cost. The eHealth actions in the Digital Agenda
  aim at empowering citizens by ensuring secure online access for citizens to their
  health data and supporting deployment of interoperable solutions for eHealth.

T. Peetso
Unit H1 – Health and Wellbeing, Directorate-General Communications Networks,
Content and Technology (DG CONNECT), European Commission, Ottawa, ON, Canada
e-mail: terje.peetso@ec.europa.eu

© Springer International Publishing Switzerland 2017
G. Rinaldi (ed.), *New Perspectives in Medical Records*, TELe-Health,
DOI 10.1007/978-3-319-28661-7_9

- The Directive on the application of patients' rights in cross-border healthcare [3] was adopted in 2011 and its Article 14 establishing the eHealth Network [4], marked a further step towards cooperation on eHealth. One of the objectives of the Network is to draw up guidelines on a non-exhaustive list of data that are to be included in patients' summaries and that can be shared between health professionals to enable continuity of care and patient safety across borders is already achieved as the guidelines on minimum/non-exhaustive patient summary data set for electronic exchange [5] were adopted in November 2013.
- The eHealth Task Force Report 'Redesigning health in Europe for 2020' [6] of May 2012 underlined the importance of access to data and data sharing while carefully implementing the requirements of data security and privacy. Among other recommendations the Task Force encouraged the integration of data into large European data sets and enhanced access for researchers.
- 'The eHealth Action Plan 2012–2020: Innovative healthcare for the 21st century' [7] consolidates the work at the EU level into four groups of activities each of which addresses the issues relevant to the development and deployment of EHR: (1) achieving wider interoperability in eHealth services; (2) supporting research, development, innovation and competitiveness in eHealth through the seventh Framework Programme, Competitiveness and Innovation Programme and the EU Framework Programme for Research and Innovation Horizon 2020 [8]; (3) facilitating uptake and ensuring wider deployment of eHealth; and (4) promoting a policy dialogue and international cooperation on eHealth at global level.
- On 10 April 2014, the European Commission published the Green Paper on mobile health [9], which is an emerging and rapidly developing field that has a growing role in data collection and data sharing for healthcare professionals and citizens. Several mHealth tools may help in accessing EHR, support data management and therefore contribute to the better health outcomes. The public consultation on the Green Paper ran for three months, and its results demonstrate that careful attention should be given to the aspects of privacy and security, patient safety, legal clarity and evidence on cost-effectiveness [10].
- The Communication from the Commission 'The Digital Single Market strategy' [11] of 6 May 2015 includes 16 initiatives to be delivered by the end of 2016. Although the strategy is aiming primarily in the completion of the Digital Single Market as one of the Commission's ten political priorities, several of its initiatives enhance eHealth directly or indirectly. Specifically, telemedicine and mHealth are mentioned under interoperability and standardisations, but work towards cybersecurity, availability of high-speed and secure infrastructures and improvement of citizens' digital skills support has an impact also on the further development and uptake of eHealth and EHR. The Commission has recently launched open consultations to gather stakeholders' views on several initiatives [12].

9.2   The eHealth Action Plan 2012–2020: Innovative Healthcare for the Twenty-First Century

The eHealth Action Plan 2012–2020 was published on 6 December 2012, and it aims at addressing barriers that hinder the implementation of 'fully mature and interoperable eHealth system in Europe'. Several actions are relevant to the EHR:

- The Action Plan recognises the need for an eHealth interoperability framework, building on eHealth roadmaps and the general European Interoperability Framework [13] with its four levels of interoperability: legal, organisational, semantic and technical. All four levels are regular and important items in the agenda of the eHealth Network.
- Under the Health Programme 2008–2013, the Commission mandated a study examining Member States' laws on electronic health records in order to make recommendations to the eHealth Network on legal aspects of interoperability. The study demonstrated that 'there are major disparities between countries on the deployment of EHRs part of an interoperable infrastructure that allows different healthcare providers to access and update health data in order to ensure the continuity of care of the patient. The same can be said about the approach taken to regulate EHRs – some countries have set specific rules for EHRs, others rely on general health records and data protection legislation' [14]. In addition to the EHRs systems and laws, the study looked at the content, interoperability and security aspects, patient consent, creation of access and update, patients' rights over the data, liability, secondary use and archiving. The final report gives recommendations at the national and the EU level.
- The research and innovation priorities are divided between short-term/midterm and long-term research priorities that include Public-Private Partnerships and Pre-Commercial Procurement and Public Procurement of Innovation for new products, scalability, interoperability and effective eHealth solutions supported by defined standards and common guidelines. Furthermore, under the European Innovation Partnership on Active and Healthy Ageing [15], special attention is given to the innovation of care for an ageing population aiming at personalised, integrated care in which integrated EHR plays a central role.
- The third part of the eHealth Action Plan lists actions facilitating uptake and ensuring wider deployment of eHealth. These actions include leveraging the Connecting Europe Facility (CEF) and the European Regional Development Fund (ERDF) for the large-scale deployment of eHealth. While the ERDF 'Elements for a Common Strategic Framework 2014–2020' [16] defines several key actions that contribute to the wider use of eHealth services in general, the funding from CEF supports more specifically cross-border exchange of health data and use of ePrescription. The Innovation and Networks Executive Agency published on 17 November 2015 calls for proposals to improve European digital services, including eHealth. A total of €17 million is available, of which €7.5 million is for eHealth Generic Services [17].

- Interoperability aspects of data sharing are also part of the international cooperation, in particular, the work with WHO and of the Memorandum of Understanding between the European Commission and the US Department of Health and Human Services signed in 2010 [18]. The objective of the Memorandum of Understanding is to accelerate progress towards widespread deployment and daily use of internationally recognised standards that support electronic health information and communication technology. Among other activities the work was supported by the FP7 funded project Trillium Bridge [19] that aimed at establishing the foundations of an interoperability bridge to meaningfully exchange patient summaries and electronic health records among the EU and the USA.

9.3 EU Projects Supporting the Implementation of the Cross-Border Exchange of Health Data

The EU has funded and continues to fund through its research and innovation programmes CIP/PSP, Public Health, FP7 and Horizon 2020 projects addressing challenges of sharing health data across the borders.

9.3.1 epSOS

The project Smart Open Services for European Patients (epSOS) [20] focussed on cross-border access to patient summary data sets and ePrescriptions and involved 25 different European countries during the course of the project. The project came to an end in June 2014 and demonstrated that it is possible to improve the quality and safety of healthcare provided to patients outside their usual country of residence, through sharing of patient health information for the purpose of receiving better and more informed treatment abroad. The project results also stressed that for achieving these objectives, a more sustainable legal framework needs to be in place.

epSOS deliverables, components and pilot infrastructure are used in projects and initiatives such as EXPAND [21], e-SENS [22], STORK 2.0 [23] (with its eHealth pilot based on epSOS infrastructure), Trillium Bridge (see above) and the eHealth Network.

9.3.2 EXPAND

Expanding Health Data Interoperability Services (EXPAND) is a Thematic Network whose 'main goal is to progress towards an environment of sustainable cross-border eHealth services, established at EU level by the Connecting Europe Facility (CEF) and at national level, through the deployment of suitable national infrastructures and services' [21].

EXPAND is supporting both the eHealth Network with information and assets and the Member States, by establishing a cooperation platform towards the upkeep of cross-border health services. The project will end on 31 December 2015 and involves 16 Member States and Switzerland.

9.4   Patients' Access to Health Data

Today, it is recognised by all stakeholders that citizen/patient should have a central role in healthcare systems. Citizen/patient empowerment is a backbone of the eHealth Action Plan 2012–2020, and the eHealth Task Force Report underlines citizen's access to their health data. However, the eHealth Stakeholder Group identified in its Report 'Patient Access to Electronic Health Records' [24] of June 2013 several obstacles in accessing EHR:

• Lack of guarantees of privacy and confidentiality
• Lack of equal access to the Internet, clarity of expectations and IT literacy
• Lack of information, trust and acceptance

The 'Overview of the national laws on electronic health records in the EU Member States' [14] indicated that among the countries that do not allow patients to access all the content of their EHRs, the typical exception is that access could cause harm to the patient. Member States have implemented different approaches to regulate the patient's access to more sensitive data, e.g. the healthcare provider may set a time limit of up to 6 months upon forwarding data to EHR, providing no direct access to the result of the examinations of diagnostic and treatment components or setting the rule requiring disclosure of information first in a meeting before being accessible on the EHR.

However, the EU project SUSTAINS [25] reported that patient associations were united in their support for implementing an array of eHealth services based on giving citizens online access to their EHR, and they did so since the beginning of the project. The patient associations strongly argued for patient choice regarding a respite of 14 days before an EHR entry is visible to the patient. They also were united in their wish to see entries immediately. The results of the project also demonstrated that the main interest of patients was reading their EHR and that the patient wanted to read everything and not just a limited version. It is important to mention that although in the beginning the project faced in one of the participating regions (Uppsala County, SE) a strong opposition from the local doctors' union towards the end of the project, the attitude was gradually changed to more positive, seeing the possibility of better communication with patients and more engagement from them.

Patient access to their health data was also addressed in the survey 'Benchmarking Deployment of eHealth among General Practitioners 2013' [26]. Overall agreement among GPs was high (76 % somewhat or strongly agreed) about the fact that the lack of a regulatory framework on confidentiality and privacy is an important barrier. GPs participating in the focus groups of the survey expressed their uneasiness about the legal grey area surrounding access to the information in existing records. The main concern was about data used by insurance companies and others, which may undermine the patient-physician trust relation.

Another project PALANTE – PAtients Leading and mANaging their healThcare through EHealth – focused on the implementation, scaling up and optimisation of seven demonstration pilots based on the concept of secure and user-friendly online access by citizens to their medical and health data [27]. The project demonstrated the importance of EHR as one of the empowerment interventions that equips patients with the capacity to participate in decisions related to their chronic disease and creates awareness. It also showed that patients who trust their healthcare system and care providers and who have a positive treatment experience are more eager to use eHealth services.

Both projects, SUSTAINS and PALANTE, underlined the importance of health literacy as it improves the understanding of information in EHR and helps patients/citizens to manage their disease and health.

9.5 Use of EHR by General Practitioners and in the EU Hospitals

According to the 'Overview of the national laws on electronic health records in the EU Member States', the EHRs are in use in all countries covered by this study. However, two surveys of 2013 – 'The European Hospital Survey: Benchmarking Deployment of eHealth Services (2012–2013)' [28] and the above-mentioned survey among GPs – are less positive demonstrating that some basic forms of EHR were in 2013 available to about 93 % of GPs and 84 % of the surveyed hospitals. Possibility to exchange medical patient data with other healthcare providers and professionals was available only for 39 % of surveyed GPs and from them less than half (49 %) used it routinely. Almost 52 % of the hospitals surveyed did not share any medical information with external general practitioners and external specialists electronically.

The General Practitioners' survey underlined that the majority of GPs place more emphasis on barriers than on benefits and identified lack of financial incentives and resources, lack of interoperability and lack of a regulatory framework on issues of confidentiality and privacy as the main barriers.

9.6 Next Steps in 2015/2016

The studies mentioned above have shown that although the situation has improved, a lot needs to be done at every level by all stakeholders involved in the process.

- The Joint Action to Support the eHealth Network (JAseHN) which is acting the main preparatory body for the eHealth Network started the work in 2015. The activities correspond to the priority areas defined in the Network's Multiannual

Work Plan 2015–2018. The next step is to put in place Connecting Europe Facility funding for shared eHealth services.

- The Horizon 2020 Work Programme 2016–2017 [29] foresees funding relevant to EHR in topics such as *SC1-PM-19–2017: PPI for uptake of standards for the exchange of digitalised healthcare records.* The proposals should aim at facilitating the uptake of newly developed solutions and focus on clear target outcomes such as allowing the sharing of health information and the use of semantically interoperable EHRs for safety alerts, decision support, care pathways or care coordination. Indirectly, information in EHRs may be relevant also for the topic *SC1-PM-18–2016: Big Data supporting Public Health policies. Topic SC1-HCO-12-2016: Digital health literacy* aims at improving citizens' understanding of online information on health and disease and increasing awareness of the opportunities of eHealth tools and enhanced skills on how to use ICT for health-related purposes.
- Following the public consultation on the Green Paper on mHealth, the Commission has launched a call for expression of interest to appoint organisations as members of a working group on mHealth assessment guidelines. The mandate of the group is to develop guidelines for assessing the validity and reliability of the data that health apps collect and process. These guidelines could be used also in the context of linking that data to the EHRs.
- As the eHealth Action Plan 2012–2020 is for 8 years but digital health is a rapidly evolving area, the Commission is currently working on the midterm evaluation for analysing the work done until 2015, updating existing actions in four areas of work of the Action Plan and bringing in new actions for addressing recent developments in the area where more in-depth actions should be taken. The public consultation for identifying concerns of all stakeholders will be launched in the first half of 2017.

Disclaimer "The views expressed in the article are the sole responsibility of the author and in no way represent the view of the European Commission and its services".

References

1. http://eur-lex.europa.eu/LexUriServ/LexUriServ.do?uri=COM:2010:2020.FIN:EN:PDF
2. http://ec.europa.eu/digital-agenda/en/digital-agenda-europe-2020-strategy
3. http://eur-lex.europa.eu/LexUriServ/LexUriServ.do?uri=OJ:L:2011:088:0045:0065:en:PDF
4. http://ec.europa.eu/health/ehealth/policy/network/index_en.htm
5. http://ec.europa.eu/health/ehealth/docs/guidelines_patient_summary_en.pdf
6. https://ec.europa.eu/digital-agenda/en/news/eu-task-force-ehealth-redesigning-health-europe-2020
7. https://ec.europa.eu/digital-agenda/en/eu-policy-ehealth
8. http://ec.europa.eu/programmes/horizon2020/en/h2020-section/health-demographic-change-and-wellbeing
9. https://ec.europa.eu/digital-agenda/en/news/green-paper-mobile-health-mhealth
10. https://ec.europa.eu/digital-agenda/en/news/mhealth-europe-preparing-ground-consultation-results-published-today
11. https://ec.europa.eu/digital-agenda/en/news/digital-single-market-strategy-europe-com2015-192-final

12. https://ec.europa.eu/digital-agenda/en/digital-me/consultations
13. http://ec.europa.eu/isa/documents/isa_annex_ii_eif_en.pdf
14. http://ec.europa.eu/health/ehealth/docs/laws_report_recommendations_en.pdf
15. http://ec.europa.eu/research/innovation-union/index_en.cfm?section=active-healthy-ageing
16. Staff Working Document SWD (2012) 61 of 14.3.2012
17. https://ec.europa.eu/inea/en/connecting-europe-facility/cef-telecom/apply-funding/
    2015-cef-telecom-call-ehealth-2015-cef-tc-2015
18. https://ec.europa.eu/digital-agenda/en/transatlantic cooperation
19. http://www.trilliumbridge.eu/
20. http://www.epsos.eu/home/about-epsos.html
21. http://www.expandproject.eu/
22. http://www.esens.eu/home/
23. https://www.eid-stork2.eu/
24. http://ec.europa.eu/digital-agenda/en/news/commission-publishes-four-reports-ehealth-stake-
    holder-group
25. Support User Access to Information and Services (SUSTAINS) http://www.sustainsproject.eu/
26. https://ec.europa.eu/digital-agenda/en/news/benchmarking-deployment-ehealth-among-gen-
    eral-practitioners-2013-smart-20110033
27. https://www.palante-project.eu/home
28. http://ec.europa.eu/digital-agenda/en/news/european-hospital-survey-benchmarking-deploy-
    ment-ehealth-services-2012-2013
29. http://ec.europa.eu/research/participants/data/ref/h2020/wp/2016_2017/main/h2020-
    wp1617-health_en.pdf

Clinical Information in Use: Problems, Outcomes and Challenges from Experience

10

Gabriele Cipriani

10.1 Broad Expectations...

eHealth is frequently presented as a remedy to solve very different problems, such as improving the quality of healthcare, increasing labour productivity by reducing absences from work, rationalising the functioning of health systems and reducing their cost, lessening social inequalities in access to care and, not least, promoting economic growth through the development of systems based on information and communication technology.

The discourse is based on the axiom that eHealth can only be good for patients and practitioners. As a result, eHealth is presented in many for a almost as an end in itself, as if the technological frontier should uncritically drive the policy choices, within a one-size-fits-all logic.

...with mixed results

After more than 20 years from its inception, results of eHealth development are however mixed. No one seems in the position to predict if and when the expectations will become reality. For example, the analysis of the literature by Piette et al. reveals that the eHealth may improve medical treatment in low- and middle-income

The opinions expressed by the author in this publication in no way commit his employer, the European Court of Auditors.

G. Cipriani
European Court of Auditors, Luxembourg, G.D., Luxembourg
e-mail: gabriele.cipriani@eca.europa.eu

countries. However, there is no sufficient evidence as regards the economic benefits and impact on patients' health.[1] Furthermore, there is no assurance (yet, a must when it comes to human health) to obtain favourable clinical outcomes in the medium and long term.

This situation has generated an expectation gap, leading to disaffection, tensions and frustrations. In short, eHealth development has created a significant market opportunity for the industry,[2] but the predicted 'revolution' in the delivery of health services has not yet materialised. Many potential users, not least including the medical profession, still need to be convinced about the positive effects of the deployment of eHealth applications. As it has been observed, 'most CIS [computerised information systems] implementations fail because, despite high investments in terms of both time and financial resources, physicians simply do not use them.'[3]

10.2 No Overall Intervention Logic…

The axiom that eHealth can only be good for patients and practitioners has legitimated in most cases public authorities to free themselves of setting up an intervention logic throwing light on a number of key questions: What is the problem? What options are available to sort it out? How overall costs compare with expected benefits? How eHealth development is going to be governed? What indicators can meaningfully measure progress?

The crucial impact of some structural preconditions has been overlooked, such as the availability of high potential networks,[4] an appropriate regulatory environment (in particular concerning the protection of personal data)[5] or the formulation of guidelines for technological development. The flourishing of uncoordinated

---

[1] See Piette JD, Lun KC, Moura LA, Fraser HSF, Mechael PN, Powell J et al., *Impacts of e-health on the outcomes of care in low- and middle-income countries: where do we go from here?*, Bull World Health Organ 2012, 90:365–372. See also Black AD., Car J., Pagliari C, Anandan C, Cresswell K, Bokun T et al., *The impact of eHealth on the quality and safety of health care: a systematic overview*, PLoS Med 2011, 8:e1000387; van Gemert-Pijnen JEWC, Wynchank S, Covvey HD, Ossebaard HC, *Improving the credibility of electronic health technologies*, Bull World Health Organ 2012, 90:323–323A; Hoerbst A, Hackl WO, Blomer R, Ammenwerth E. *The status of IT service management in health care – ITIL(R) in selected European countries*. BMC medical informatics and decision making. 2011;11:76. PubMed PMID: 22189035. Pubmed Central PMCID: 3276449.

[2] The estimated value of the ICT systems market in the health field is about €60 billion, of which one third in Europe.

[3] Rodríguez, C and Pozzebon, M, *A Paradoxical World: Exploring the Discursive Construction of Collaboration in a Competitive Institutional Context*. In 11th APROS Colloquium (4–7 December 2005), Melbourne, 2006: 306–320. Cited by Greenhalgh T et al., *Adoption and non-adoption of a shared electronic summary record in England: a mixed-method case study*, BMJ 2010;340:c3111.

[4] OECD Internet Economy Outlook 2012, p. 201.

[5] The right to protection of personal data is explicitly recognised by EU law. It is based on the principle that the use of personal data shall be subject to the consent of the person concerned.

initiatives has resulted in a 'patchwork' of IT systems which, in turn, has hindered the capacity of mutual interaction.[6] Also, once the systems were made operational, there has been often a lack of capacity to manage them, leading to unexpected costs, reduced use of applications and users' dissatisfaction.[7] The one-size-fits-all approach has failed to take account of local differences concerning the level of healthcare and users' digital health literacy. This demonstrates that to fulfil its full potential, eHealth requires also a permanent cultural adaptation. Indeed, 'a 'technically best' system can be brought to its knees by people who have low psychological ownership in the system and who vigorously resist its implementation'.[8] Furthermore, large-scale ICT systems 'need to be managed over time as use may be transformed into non-use, resources initially gained may be later lost, and collaboration with key stake-holders may turn into conflict'.[9]

…many actors…

eHealth development is characterised by a multiplicity of stakeholders (hospitals, public health authorities, medical profession, systems' managers, industry), each of them having a good reason to intervene in this field. Against this background, the absence of intervention logic discussed earlier has produced a 'Babel tower' effect, both semantic (What is eHealth in practice? Who is supposed to benefit primarily? Can any application be an eHealth tool?) and decisional/organisational (Who decides what? How is the development process governed?).

One should also note the lack of a clear sharing of roles between EU countries (that are responsible for the organisation and the management of the health system) and the European Union (that holds a complementary role).[10] An assessment of the general value of EU-level public health actions over the last 20 years resulted in mainly ambivalent judgments. The EU has strengthened in general its role. The establishment of EU-level agencies dealing with public health topics is considered positive. Successes in smoking prohibition, food safety and infectious disease control are also acknowledged. It is mainly thanks to the EU that thousands of researchers and practitioners can interact and exchange experiences among them. However, the available evidence of the impact of EU health policies, infrastructure and actions seems elusive. In particular, the assurance of health protection in European policies

---

[6] OECD Internet Economy Outlook 2012, p. 15, 210. For example, in Italy, where the management of healthcare is a competence of the regions, eHealth development has been started in any order, in the absence of Health Ministry's guidelines. This has required a process of ex post adjustment for the regions having already put in place eHealth applications.

[7] van Gemert-Pijnen JEWC et al., op. cit.

[8] Lorenzi NM, Riley RT. *Managing change: an overview*, Journal of the American Medical Informatics Association Volume 7, Number 2, Mar/Apr 2000, p. 116.

[9] Constantinides, P, Barrett, M. *Large-Scale ICT Innovation, Power and Organizational Change: The Case of a Regional Health Information Network*, Journal of Applied Behavioral Science 2006; Vol. 42 No. 1, March 2006, p. 89.

[10] See Articles 6, 9 and 168 of the Treaty on the Functioning of the European Union.

is perceived as a missed opportunity.[11] Assessments of the EU Health programmes criticise missing prioritisation of topics and identification of how the results will produce the intended impacts.[12] Also, duplication and overlap have been noted between, for example, the Health Programme and the Framework Programme for Research and Innovation.[13]

… risking to lose sight of patients

The combination of a lack of intervention logic and the plurality of stakeholders has given de facto the leadership to those with the strongest capacity to impose their vested interests.[14] This has resulted in a prevailing 'offer'-driven rather than 'need'-oriented approach, focussed on applying to healthcare technological solutions developed for other purposes and objectives. Following this logic, eHealth becomes merely a product to which the user must adapt (and not the other way round).[15] Such approach is in fact aimed at 'customers' rather than 'patients', thus denying in substance the individual character of the application of the clinical method. Hence, the patient looks as the weak ring of the chain, like an earthen vessel thrown amidst iron jars.

10.3   Towards eHealth Resetting

The above indicates the need to a fundamental rethinking of eHealth's role in the society and its 'architectural' setup. Three main drivers of change can be identified.

10.3.1 Pulling in the Same Direction: A Strategic Approach

To improve efficiency and mitigate the risk of duplication and overlapping actions, the establishment at European level of a comprehensive strategy for eHealth should define intervention fields and specific objectives, on the basis of member states' and EU respective roles and responsibilities.

---

[11] Rosenkötter N, Clemens T, Sørensen K, Brand H, Twentieth anniversary of the European Union health mandate: taking stock of perceived achievements, failures and missed opportunities – a qualitative study, BMC Public Health 2013, 13:1074.

[12] European Court of Auditors. The European Union's Public Health Programme (2003–2007): An effective way to improve health?, Special Report No 2//2009. Luxembourg, 2009.

[13] European Commission, Mid-term evaluation of the Health Programme 2008–2013, SWD (2012) 83 final, Brussels, 29.3.2012, p. 13–14.

[14] Rosenkötter N, Clemens T, Sørensen K, Brand H, op. cit., note the need for strong partnerships to counter strong industrial lobbying groups. They refer to analyses made by Greer SL, Hervey TK, Mackenbach JP, McKee M. *Health law and policy in the European union*. Lancet. 2013; 381(9872):1135–1144; Buchner B. *Nutrition, obesity and EU health policy*. Eur J Health Law. 2011; 18(1):1–8; McKee M. *A European alcohol strategy*. BMJ. 2006; 333(7574):871–872.

[15] van Gemert-Pijnen JEWC et al., op. cit.

Due to its far-reaching implications for the quality and the modalities of delivering healthcare services, such strategy should be patient-centred and involve co-design and co-development with the medical profession.

10.3.2 Addressing Patients' Needs Effectively: Action Based on Convincing Clinical Results

eHealth should promote long-term value-based healthcare innovation. It should address public health as well as medical science ensuring patient empowerment.

As a tool supporting patients' care, eHealth applications should undergo the same precautionary process applicable to pharmaceuticals products. The effectiveness in healthcare of such applications should therefore be assessed and ascertained before their use, for example, through pilot projects.

10.3.3 Making Decision Makers Accountable: Analysis of Costs and Benefits

As for any public intervention funded with taxpayers' money, eHealth's investments should undergo a proper analysis of costs and benefits. Such analysis should extend beyond the direct financial impact and include in particular societal values, such as reduced admission and time spent in care institutions and improved interactions between patients and carers.

Public authorities should be able to justify the choices made and report about the results expected and those actually achieved.

Bibliography

1. Black AD, Car J, Pagliari C, Anandan C, Cresswell K, Bokun T et al (2011) The impact of eHealth on the quality and safety of health care: a systematic overview. PLoS Med 8:e1000387
2. Buchner B (2011) Nutrition, obesity and EU health policy. Eur J Health Law 18(1):1–8
3. Catwell L, Sheikh A (2009) Evaluating eHealth interventions: the need for continuous systemic evaluation. PLoS Med 6(8):e1000126. doi:10.1371/journal.pmed.1000126
4. Cipriani G (2010) The EU budget, responsibility without accountability? Ceps, Brussels
5. European Commission (2012) eHealth Task Force Report – redesigning health in Europe for 2020, Luxembourg
6. European Commission, Mid-term evaluation of the Health Programme 2008–2013, SWD (2012) 83 final, Brussels, 29.3.2012
7. European Commission, eHealth Action Plan 2012–2020, COM (2012) 736, Brussels, 6.12.2012
8. Constantinides, P, Barrett M (2006) Large-scale ICT innovation, power and organizational change: the case of a Regional Health Information Network. J Appl Behav Sci 42(1):76–90
9. European Court of Auditors (2009) The European Union's Public Health Programme (2003–2007): an effective way to improve health? Special report no 2//2009, Luxembourg
10. Gaddi AV, Manca M (2014) Capello F: eHealth, care and quality of life. Springer, Milan, Italy

11. Greer SL, Hervey TK, Mackenbach JP, McKee M (2013) Health law and policy in the European union. Lancet 381(9872):1135–1144
12. Greenhalgh T et al (2010) Adoption and non-adoption of a shared electronic summary record in England: a mixed-method case study. BMJ 340:c3111
13. Hoerbst A, Hackl WO, Blomer R, Ammenwerth E (2011) The status of IT service management in health care – ITIL(R) in selected European countries. BMC Med Inform Decis Mak 11:76, Pubmed Central PMCID: 3276449
14. Lorenzi NM, Riley RT (2000) Managing change: an overview. J Am Med Inform Assoc 7(2): 116–124
15. Mair FS, May C, O'Donnell C, Finch T, Sullivan F, Murray E (2012) Factors that promote or inhibit the implementation of e-health systems: an explanatory systematic review. Bull World Health Organ 90:357–364
16. McKee M (2006) A European alcohol strategy. BMJ 333(7574):871–872
17. McLoughlin I, Wilson R, Martin M (2013) Digital government @ work – a social informatics perspective. Oxford University Press, Oxford
18. OECD (2012) Internet economy outlook, Paris
19. Piette JD, Lun KC, Moura LA, Fraser HSF, Mechael PN, Powell J et al (2012) Impacts of e-health on the outcomes of care in low- and middle-income countries: where do we go from here? Bull World Health Organ 90:365–372
20. Robertson A, Cresswell K, Takian A, Petrakaki D, Crowe S, Cornford T et al (2010) Implementation and adoption of nationwide electronic health records in secondary care in England: qualitative analysis of interim results from a prospective national evaluation. BMJ 341:c4564, Pubmed Central PMCID: 2933355
21. Rodríguez, C Pozzebon MA Paradoxical world: exploring the discursive construction of collaboration in a competitive institutional context. In 11th APROS Colloquium (4–7 December 2005), Melbourne, 2006: 306–320
22. Rosenkötter N, Clemens T, Sørensen K, Brand H (2013) Twentieth anniversary of the European Union health mandate: taking stock of perceived achievements, failures and missed opportunities – a qualitative study. BMC Public Health 13:1074
23. Rinaldi G, Capello F, Gaddi A (2014) Medical data, information economy and federative networks: the concepts underlying the comprehensive electronic clinical record framework. Nova Science Publisher, New York
24. Touré H. In: The bigger picture for e-health, Bull World Health Organ 2012, 90: 330–33112-040512
25. van Gemert-Pijnen JEWC, Wynchank S, Covvey HD, Ossebaard HC (2012) Improving the credibility of electronic health technologies. Bull World Health Organ 90:323–323A

Medical Records, eHealth and Health IT: What Are the Key Points for the Organizational Benefits and for the Improvements of the Modern Local Health Organisations?

11

Franco Falcini and Giovanni Rinaldi

11.1 Introduction

The use of ICT disciplines in health is dealing with a grave underestimation of organizational problems. Thus, the ICT approach that seemed an organizational way for saving money in some cases did not lead to expected results [1]. The expectations of patients and caregivers did not correspond to their experiences of the use of Internet-based applications for self-care: in fact, while patients would be supported in solving their health problems, caregivers are worried about medico-legal concerns. However, the applications failed to support self-care because eHealth is more than just a technological intervention [2]. The trend, in fact, is to drastically separate the technical functions with the health commitment or health needs, with the organisational activities, while a coproduction approach seems more appropriate in terms of information set treatment for multi-agency activities [3]. The multi-agency care and the contexts in which shared technical infrastructure and new working practices are being constructed have the following characteristics: the users belong to different agencies and they also have different groups of value, priorities and perspectives of practitioners, managers, technicians and clients or patients; the nature of health and social care relationships produces issues of practice's governance and essential information, and these are issues of responsibility which cannot be reduced to simple functions or expressed in terms of simple function. The only level represented is the operational one, while the organisational and control levels are often missing. Every characteristic means that any approach to rationality in design or communication has to be preceded by, and be a consequence of, shared

F. Falcini
Azienda USL, Romagna, Italy

G. Rinaldi (✉)
Ospedali Riuniti Marche Nord, Pesaro, Italy
e-mail: rinaldi8giovanni@gmail.com

© Springer International Publishing Switzerland 2017
G. Rinaldi (ed.), *New Perspectives in Medical Records*, TELe-Health,
DOI 10.1007/978-3-319-28661-7_11

sense making just as the products of these processes (technical and organisational systems) must themselves be "made sense of" through use and governance. It is because there is a cultural gap between the requirements and the technological implementation: this gap can be cancelled promoting specific learning programmes at higher education, but this is not enough: the coproduction in the developing of health system in the implementation phase is fundamental.

11.2   Policies for the Implementation of the Health Information System in Large Healthcare Organisations

The information system is universally considered as a lever for change.

During the phases of implementation, it is influenced by actions fostering the implementation pushing innovative actions, but it is also affected by actions that hinder it.

The phases of implementation regard the strategic change, the organisational change and the change management that depends on the features (width, time and depth), administration of power (choice of key persons and strategic alliances) and organisational levers (organisation of the technical management, planning and control).

The most recent organisational theories regarding the design and implementation of information systems claim that the planning of the organisation and the design of information systems are two activities that coincide.

Moreover, the strategic characteristics of the company's information system support the revision of organisational processes; the empowerment of skills and the role of employees within the organization and the revision of the mechanisms of power. In healthcare it is primary that the transversal role is assigned to the information system as the main instrument of integration.

But organizations are "open environments", i.e., they interact with the environment and are affected by it; there is no system/organizational absolute best, but one that fits better to the specific current situation determined by the environment in which the organization is operating.

Organising means being able to fit to the external environment and to the new requirements that it imposes on organizations. In this context, information systems play an important role as they can and must contribute to support the organizational flexibility that the company needs to adapt to their sphere of activity through the provision of integrated information.

In this context we identify three operational blocks.

The first at a low level is connected to the operational activities. It deals with the control processes daily used in the execution of activities and specific tasks. It needs more detailed information.

The second (the middle layer) is about the control of management. It is connected to the implementation of the policies and the strategies in order to reach goals. It valuates and provides detailed information in order to address the policies and the behaviours of actors in the organisational process.

At a higher level the third block is the management of the company. It is connected to the strategic planning. It needs synthetic and precise information and comparison with other institutions.

In this traditional, pyramidal, three-layer architecture, each layer has its own software procedures and applications.

The level of operating procedures is composed by software application managing (the health departments, the booking of the health services, stock management and order procedures) and by longitudinal services (laboratory information system, radiological information system, the integrated management of the clinical images (PACS) and the management of operating rooms). The first level provides data that will be used by the upper levels which have a purpose of government.

This traditional vision we have depicted is complete with the layer allowing the exchange of data with external organisations. The middleware has the aim to extract data I need to exchange from the internal database, translate data in a form negotiated with the destination, send data and also in opposite direction from external sources towards the own information system.

The middleware, allowing the data exchange, has also the important aim to allow the vision of clinical documents to the patient.

Obviously this opportunity is fostered by the implementation of different electronic patient records and/or a whole clinical data repository.

At last the recent improvements in technology and the advent of the personal devices like smartphones have requested to reinforce the layer dedicated to the external communication with the production of portal and apps.

Employers and patients can access to the portal and to the apps in order to use some services of the information system.

We know that these concepts were not always supported by adequate technological deployment. Especially in Italy, the computerisation of local health organisations and hospitals is preceded by the implementation of individual technological islands connected by middleware. This sort of implementation has shown great problems in organisations.

However, the implementation of enterprise resource plannings (ERPs) in the health context is often based on the ERP born for industrial or commercial environment.

Enterprise resource planning, or ERP, is a type of integrated management software that allows an organisation to use a system of integrated applications in order to manage the business. ERP software integrates all facets of an operation, including development, manufacturing, sales and marketing. In the health context the ERP includes the electronic patient record (EPR) enabled for each department.

The typical modules included are the following:

- Patient management (appointments, registration, admission, discharge and transfer)
- Financial management (accounts payable, accounts receivable, general ledger and fixed assets)
- Materials management (inventory and purchase)
- Human resource (scheduling, training and payroll)

- Ancillary services (dietary, laboratory and pharmacy)
- Management information (reporting on and providing statistics on various issues)

In the healthcare context, these modules are integrated with specific modules for the management of the clinical data: medical records.

Traditionally electronic patient records are modules used in each clinical department in order to manage clinical data collected in different encounters.

They manage the entire episode (from admission to discharge) with a peculiar focus on the clinical data.

Given the pervasiveness of ERP system, the EPR is often poor of functionality related to clinical data management. This is an important issue to keep in mind because clinicians need to use effective medical records and not only general pervasive functions devoted more to administrative issues rather than clinical ones.

This is a key issue reported by clinicians, and technicians tend to overcome it by proposing specific medical records interconnected to the infrastructure.

Anyhow a longitudinal layer offering medical services is provided by ERPs: LIS, RIS, PACS and operating rooms.

Ideally the implementation of an ERP in the health context responds to a mix of motivations:

- Technological performance
  - Search for IT integration
  - Improve IT infrastructure capabilities
  - Modernise IT systems
  - Improve IT productivity
  - Build a knowledge management infrastructure
- Managerial – operational
  - Improve effectiveness of administrative processes
  - Improve administrative data availability and accessibility
  - Improve HR management performance
  - Improve administrative data accuracy and relevance
  - Search for business process integration
- Clinical – operational
  - Improve effectiveness and efficiency of patient care
  - Improve effectiveness of clinical processes
  - Facilitate access to clinical information
  - Improve patient safety
  - Enhance the preservation of patients' privacy
- Managerial – strategic
  - Improve administrative performance management capabilities
  - Enhance compliance with laws and regulations
  - Support organisational growth and expansion
  - Facilitate connectivity with major stakeholders
  - Improve decision-making processes
- Clinical – strategic
  - Strengthen clinical strategic positioning
  - Transform care delivery and respond to changing need

- Improve clinical performance management capabilities
- Implement a patient safety culture
- Financial performance
  - Monitor cost trends
  - Increase profitability or return on investment
  - Improve financial transparency
  - Monitor asset value

Very often, it is worth noting that there is a clear domination of motivations related to managerial performance over clinical performance: improving the effectiveness of the administrative process rather than improving the effectiveness and efficiency of care provided to patients is the leverage for the implementation of ERP.

This is known as top-down implementation and it is often rejected by clinicians. They prefer to choose medical record tools rather than the systems that could impose administrative control also.

Medical professionals prefer to maintain their control.

As a consequence, the ERP tends to create a conflict between managerial and medical rationalities. ERPs are a set of integrated modules, and it is practically impossible to avoid the control over the organisation. However, both sets of definitive stakeholders realised that eventually consensus on the objectives and scope of the ERP had to be reached. This meant that managerial and medical rationalities had to come together in a mutually acceptable manner.

This gap depends on the methodology used for promoting the ERP in the health organisation.

We must not forget that the implementation of a pervasive information system is not only a technological matter but, since it involves people, it has a social component: it is a sociotechnical system.

While knowing the problems manifested by the introductions of ERP systems in the health context, for example, in the UK where the top-down implementation has caused disaffection and "do not use", in environments where currently the "island model" (such as in Italy) prevails, the ERP implementation could be the first step for enhancing the awareness that a pervasive information system can be favourable both for administrative staff and for clinicians.

We want to emphasise that the implementation of a complex pervasive system must be done according to the co-production rule in which all the actors are involved in a mutual make sense.

11.3   Medical Records Inside Organisations

Medical record systems are described by literature in different ways: they range from the model that offers only a specialist point of view up to the collection of the all medical events in the life of the individuals.

We want to emphasise that this is not only a clinical vision; the correct organisation of clinical data is fundamental also for planning services, for epidemiological analysis and for managerial aims. For these reasons medical records cannot be the only tools for doctors (which remain the main users).

Medical records respond to the requests done by the professionals, who need clinical information to execute clinical actions.

But also the requirements of the patients in some cases must be answered, according to doctors and stakeholders. Moreover, the information of individuals are treated also for epidemiological analysis, national surveillance or medical research.

These considerations suggest that medical records do not have to be a static object like a mere collection of static informatics artefacts but a set of information reachable by professionals who need to consume the information according to their role.

Both literature and practice have shown a great amount of models that reflect the specific requirements done by specialists or GPs.

We know that literature proposes different classifications especially based on a medical specialist. This is correct, but inevitably partial from a comprehensive point of view. They claim to be complete for the specific purpose of caring of the individuals in the specific episode.

Moreover, we don't have to forget that the inclusion of genetic data requires some times in modern medicine.

As we have seen, the clinical organisation requires the management of different medical records for different aims. In hospital departments, they generally respond to the management of the episode of care, whereas GPs manage the data in a more comprehensive way. Furthermore RIS, PACS and LIS provide data from instrumental investigation.

Moreover, we know that patients want to have access to their data. The patient requires a longitudinal care record in which all clinical data collected in different episode must be stored. Doctors and stakeholders promote the empowering of the patient not only to allow him access to his data but asking the same patient to interact in specific health spaces providing useful information in the disease care processes. And they do, as they browse the Internet, collect information and discuss with other patients about their pathologies.

And, at last, the medical research requires its own medical record system, connected with practice or with the patient lifestyle, in order to make the research done reliable.

The traditional classifications of the medical records based on the nature of the information collected are useful for organisational purposes. These visions designed to classify the information are correct because they answer the question "what are the information that have been generated?" and "which information do we need for caring people?".

They reveal the complex nature of the clinical information and promote a conception of medical records in which the tools for consuming such information are provided together with tools for collecting information.

Another element that generates complexity is the vision of the shared medical information.

But the complexity of the system and the nature of the medical records – a living complex object feed by different actors and accessible by different stakeholders and by the patient – require a more complete vision.

Medical profession is a collaborative work engaging different actors (including the patient) belonging to different organisations and perspectives but acting, often, on the same information, with the aim to create a virtual community in which the actors collect information, make it available and seek data and services to treating it.

And this last assertions characterize the medical record systems not only as a container of information but also as a shared entry point in which services and functions are used for treating medical information, producing knowledge at the same time.

Whereas traditional hospital information systems are based on a methodology for which data are incorporated in the functions that manage them, it seems more appropriate to separate the clinical data from the functions needed for accessing, managing and treating them. These features, already proposed by CEN [4] and OpenEHR [5], should be designed within the overall systems managing the clinical pathway.

In this vision clinical data are narrowly connected to the context of the information, while the surrounding are fundamental for a better understanding, use and share of the information. Clinical data are stored in the clinical data item.

The clinical data item represents the minimal indivisible unit of information the clinician wants to record; this is collected and defined in the clinical pathway.

Clinical data items can be represented by a number of informational objects: identifiers, codes, numbers including proportions or intervals, time, date, also expressed in different units; but also by texts composed in different meanings or with different headings; different multimedia objects, objects referenced by link or pieces of information extracted by or referenced in Internet-based applications like blogs, social networks, etc.

Data item has peculiar characteristics: persistency, concerning the durability of data item; consistency, dealing with the correctness of the transaction according to rules and limits; traceability, concerning auditing information and committal; and un-cancellability, assuring that committed data are indelible in order to support future research purposes or medico-legal investigation [6].

Logically, data items are depending on basic information that make the meaning explicit, for example, unit of measure, method for treating information, clinical guidelines and medical concepts, context information (where, when, who, etc.), composition rules in order to compose information, extraction rules, privacy and consent rule, version, external data reference and metadata.

This design of structured data is flexible and opens new opportunities.

We need to overcome the traditional idea done by silos of data towards a vision of shared information.

11.4 Healthcare and Social Care Integration

We have explored the opportunity offered by the technology for the implementation of an overall integrated system in which both clinical and administrative features are provided.

This responds to a request done by administrative staff in order to manage the functions of the organisation.

Whereas the previous system was designed inside the organisation, it is frequent that the same needs are expressed by a set of organisations that must handle the same environment.

As an example, let's have a look at the workflow regarding the social care and healthcare; it is an important example of mixed actions offered by a set of organisations needing an integrated infrastructure in which information can be shared. The landscape here depicted is typical in Italy.

Healthcare and social care are closely related for the elderly, and the system proposed is mainly proposed for the elderly.

The infrastructure for the management of the social care and healthcare is a peculiar example of integration in which actions made in different organisations (medical centres, hospitals, social departments of the municipalities, private social agencies, etc.) are combined.

Each agency has its own peculiarities, it is governed by its own managers and it is part of the path, offering its own services integrated and composed with others and proposed by other agencies.

The health services are generally coordinated by the local health organisation acting on the territory and acquire services from the medical centres, hospitals, GPs and municipalities of the territory; they often require the integration with social services as part of the pathway.

Also independent social services are provided by social departments and a private sector. They are requested autonomously by the patients, but for a complete evaluation of the social and health state of the patient, it is necessary that the outcomes could be evaluated jointly.

The technical infrastructure is configured as an integrated suite that collects the workflows for the social care and healthcare.

The aim is to provide one single centre which coordinates the actions and shares social and health information, including the management of activities and the budget.

One of the difficulties in the implementation of a suite for the management of socio-sanitary activities concerns the interconnection of services between different agencies and between private companies engaged in service delivery. Generally we tend to computerise various business segments for each institution, leaving the so-called interoperability of systems for the exchange of information. This mode suffers too often from several problems mainly due to the still poor computerisation of these services by different entities.

In order to solve the problems of poor mechanisation of some services and solve problems related to the information exchange, the way of activation of a complete suite is frequently chosen, to which also external agencies can have access.

We note that in the current organisational configuration of services, they are often fragmented along different organisations, both public and private.

It is therefore necessary that both government and control (and the social and clinical management with them) can have a comprehensive view of the activities and of the services provided to patients, in order not to replicate activities and to know the detailed spending.

The suite therefore aims to manage the social and health activities in an integrated manner, allowing different agencies and public and private companies engaged in the provision of care to have a single point where the information (administrative, social and medical records) is stored and a series of functions that act on that information base.

Every institution and company can access the functionalities dedicated to it with the intention of providing services to the patient.

In order to know the comprehensive state of the patient, they can have access to all or part of the information of the patients, according to the privacy rules associated to the different operators.

This opportunity allows to choose the better services to offer to the patient.

At the same time, each task is defined by a cost so as the budget assigned to the services and also to patients.

Each time a service is provided, the cost is subtracted from the budget so you know in real time the costs incurred.

11.4.1 The Features of the Healthcare and Social Care Technical System

The main features are as follows.

- Medical and social care records, single and integrated. So that each agency enters information about its own activity during the workflow of care. This allows to create an information system where each department, according to the privacy rules, can access and check the status of the patients, without duplicating information and thus choosing the best activities to be provided.
- Workflow describing the path of each service. The complexity of services and in some cases the participation of various institutions and companies to the same services require a service orchestration in which every step of the pathway has to be defined in detail with the information that should be taken; a mode in which the step is terminated must be defined and the next one must be activated. Such step must be well defined by an operator who assumes the responsibilities. The nature of the problem addressed requires the possibility of establishing new services throughout the years; next to a series of services which become standardised, they can be specialised over time. The tool for the design and development of new workflows is one of the main features of the system; the feature must take into account the actors involved, the responsibility, the information that must be collected, the rules for the passage to the next step.
- Booking services. The feature is responsible for booking services in which the working team necessary for the execution of the services and for each of them the availability of resources over time are described. Each action taken for the patient is booked under the rules of service. In this case also, the working team

is often composed by mixed skills (doctors, nurses, social workers, etc.), and each of them is part of the budget attached to their company.

- Budget management functions. The system must allow the definition of the costs for each service. It is essential to provide the function that allows the proposed budget allocation for service and for the patient, the final allocation of the budget and the decrease of it every time the services are provided. The management of the standard cost and the final cost for the service, with associated functions of recalculation of the standard cost depending on the services provided in the last year, might be useful but not even essential.
- Data integration and verification of the services provided to the patient. Each user that must provide services to the patient can access the system and consult social and medical information useful for the services (according to the privacy rules). He can add further information and data according to the services he is providing. In this way the wealth of information of the patient increases and becomes useful for each actor. This pervasiveness of information allows to carry out checks on the adequacy of the services offered.
- Administrative functions in order to propose and fill supply contracts with the private agencies involved in the assistance of the patients.

In addition to the traditional functions of a multi-agency information system, tools dedicated to the patient empowerment and the monitoring of health status through telemedicine devices are provided.

- The patient and his family's portal. This is a key issue related to the opportunity for the patient to access his/her own clinical and social information, consult other patient suffering from the same pathology, search social and charity agencies in order to receive assistance and communicate with the stakeholders. In this case it is necessary to offer user-friendly solutions in order to make the functions to the patients accessible; the traditional way to provide the same clinical note provided by clinicians for the clinicians (e.g. the PDF referrals or medical notes) is not appropriate and useful.
- The patient summary. Extraction of synthetic data for emergency events accessible by the emergency unit.
- GP access to the social and clinical repository. GPs and also clinicians or specialists can benefit from access to social and clinical data of patients.
- Telemedicine devices integrated to the system. Telemedicine devices can be offered to the patients for monitoring the health state; this opportunity is useful for patients suffering of chronic disease. The data must be integrated with the medical record.

11.5   The eHealth Solutions

Next to the traditional solutions such as ERP, other solutions are appearing from Web 2.0. In Web 2.0– Health 2.0 – are enhanced the concepts linked to the collaboration issues, pervasive knowledge in the health context, access to personal information, open source and free innovation.

These concepts are not always separated by traditional ERP issue.

Software industries [7] are thinking to reinvent the information systems for the companies based on the new paradigms that Web 2.0 has brought, promoting collaboration between employers through social-application tools such as blogs, wikis, folksonomies, crowdsourcing, mash-ups and rich Internet applications believing that the improvement of internal and external communication could bring a significant impact on the enterprise [8].

Social services provided inside the organisations bring people together, allow the locating of expertise from across the organisation and tagging any resources to grow productivity, participation and innovation.

The clinical record systems are becoming the core application in any eHealth environment and cannot be separated by this environment because they produce the base information for each eHealth function or application or service.

eHealth solutions imply the concept of reviewing the architecture and infrastructure, in which the concepts of collaboration and sharing are enhanced.

Collaboration between stakeholders and engagement of the patient are interesting concepts to take into consideration if they are inscribed into the governance rules and provided that the privacy of the patient is made safe.

We know that these new technologies can bring improvement in the health context, but they must be governed and inscribed in the overall system.

The aim is to make the clinical information and the services needed for its fruition available.

These considerations are based on the assumption that the concepts of collaboration, sharing and pervasive knowledge must be made explicit in the architecture, fostered by the architecture.

This implies the design of an architecture set on opening, in which the collaboration functions are made explicit.

Functional services produce structured messaging and publication services capable of delivering virtual records which are assembled and presented according to the roles, rights and clinical or research situations and are available in order to be deployed, used, consumed, managed and governed.

Sharing is made real through the availability of contents which may reside in databases for structured information or can be spread in different silos of data.

But the access to that information is possible according to the user-oriented content in which contents and functionalities are assembled dynamically, locally and flexibly to meet immediate needs. It requires a significant and different conceptualization and implies complete and strong information governance.

Maintaining separate data and functions, it is useful to share clinical information: the clinical data (both information services and the contents they offer) are annotated with further data that relate to provenance, consents and purposes.

Conclusions

The key motivations that underlie the adoption of ERP systems in healthcare organisations are not only technical or administrative.

We need a new approach in the design and implementation of ICT projects, and the design and implementation cannot be a matter only for technicians.

Technicians, designers, users, doctors, patients and sponsors all must be empowered to be participants and to formulate their contributions in the process.

They cannot be divided into experts and clients: the complexity of the problem we are approaching must be considered also by a sociotechnical point of view. This new approach must be supported by specific technical tools in order to make clear the choices to provide electronic delivery of health services.

Medical records, accessible by patients, must not be only a mere list of PDF files but also a catalogue of functions where the doctor-patient relationship is made explicit and where other components creating significant healthcare value must be included.

In that, clinical information must lead to a value added in the healthcare; so some pathologies must be monitored in different ways and the involvement of the patient must be different. In this way the opportunity for the patient to be an active part in the care process can be reached. This request is reached using specific functions that enable definite information channels with appropriate professionals when certain symptoms arise according specific guidelines.

Moreover, a more user-friendly visualisation of clinical information is needed. It does not seem useful for the patient to access clinical documents compiled by clinicians for the clinicians; it is necessary to present clinical data to the patient in a comprehensible way.

Currently clinical information suffers from the managerial and administrative impositions; it is stored in DB silos, and when it is exchanged, the sense for which it was recorded is often lost, and moreover accuracy and reliability are limited.

A vision concerning the separation between clinical data and the functions needed for managing and treating them seems more useful for the purposes of sharing clinical information and collaborative activities.

References

1. Wilson C No hospital savings with electronic record: U.S. study, http://www.reuters.com/article/idUSTRE5AJ0MQ20091120
2. Nijland N, van Gemert-Pijnen J, Boer H, Steehouder M, Seydel E (2008) Evaluation of internet-based technology for supporting self-care: problems encountered by patients and caregivers when using self-care applications. J Med Internet Res 10(2):e13
3. Manatiopoulos G, McLoughlin I, Wilson R, Martin M (2009) Developing virtual healthcare systems in complex multi-agency service settings: the OLDES project. Electronic J e-Government 7 (2):163–170
4. http://www.centc251.org
5. http://www.openEHR.org
6. Rinaldi G, Gaddi A, Capello A (2013) Medical data, information economy and federative networks: the concepts underlying the co prehensive electronic clinical record framework. Hauppage NY 11788-3619. Nova Science Publishers p 1–396, ISBN: 978-1-62257-845-0
7. Oracle Publication (2009) Content management and portals. Oracle and IDG Global Solutions
8. Accenture publication. A Web 2.0 Primer. 2007 Accenture

Disease Registry: A Tool for European Cross-Border Medicine

12

Luca Sangiorgi and Marina Mordenti

12.1   What Is the Cross-Border Medicine?

The number of patients that prefer to move cross-border for diagnosis and treatment is still little and a huge amount of European citizens is addressing to national structures and local providers for healthcare issues. Nevertheless, people crossing European borders to solve issues related to health started long ago, and the trend is increasing exponentially every year.

Due to this growing movement of persons, the European Commission has been focusing its attention on cross-border medicine for more than 40 years.

As a matter of fact, the Council Regulation no. 1408 of 14 June 1971[1] approaches for the first time the application of schemes to employed persons and their families moving within the community. Starting from that regulation, the European Commission, the Parliament, and the Council of Ministers have been discussing and regulating "by legislative steps" the actions and arrangements to solve outstanding issues, aiming at providing a European legal framework to member states. In fact, from June 1971 to date, a lot of legal documents have been produced to formalize care and treatment in case of patients, medical staff, and nurse personnel that decided to move as *transfrontalier*.

The conclusive action of this complex, convoluted and long *iter*, is the Directive 2011/24/EU of the European Parliament and of the Council, dated 9 March 2011, on the application of patients' rights in cross-border healthcare and the relative

---

[1] Regulation (EEC) No 1408/71 of the Council of 14 June 1971 on the application of social security schemes to employed persons and their families moving within the community. Official Journal of the European Communities, 1971; L149/2.

L. Sangiorgi (✉) • M. Mordenti
CLIBI – SSD Genetica Medica, Istituto Ortopedico Rizzoli, Bologna, Italy
e-mail: luca.sangiorgi@ior.it

© Springer International Publishing Switzerland 2017
G. Rinaldi (ed.), *New Perspectives in Medical Records*, TELe-Health,
DOI 10.1007/978-3-319-28661-7_12

transposition into national law in 2013.[2] The first sentence of Article 1 clarifies the main subject of the Directive: "This Directive provides rules for facilitating the access to safe and high-quality cross-border healthcare and promotes cooperation on healthcare between Member States, in full respect of national competencies in organising and delivering healthcare."

This Directive aims at regulating many aspects of mobility, solving borderline and ambiguous mechanisms related to patients' rights and entitlements providing clear and reliable rules. Moreover, it aims at defining financial procedures, reimbursing actions and patient accessibility to avoid potential problems for healthcare providers.

Even if there is a lack of information flows due, for example, to existing differences among European countries in healthcare systems or procedures, the Directive 2011/24/EU unravels information (a) to define rules to simplify access to safe and high-quality cross-border medicine, (b) to guarantee patient mobility in Europe, (c) to increase coworking in healthcare scenario between member countries, and (d) to achieve the "continuity of care" principle.

12.1.1 The Nature of Being Mobile

The term "mobility" across European countries is frequently unclear and has a broad meaning because it refers to various distant scenarios. To a preliminary evaluation, mobility indicates "a patient that moves to a foreign country for a specific treatment."

But the mobility that for sure engages patients involves also healthcare professionals, partnerships, data, health services, and many sub-aspects of the mentioned features. In this light, not only patients move from home to other European countries to receive care but also medical doctors and nurses go abroad for training, for specific research projects, to provisionally provide services or to establish their long-term job in another European member state.

In addition, some services are *transfrontalier* by nature, for example, the transfusion system, blood facility, or tissue and cell transplantation service. But the list of mobile prospects can be increased considering particular services of eHealth, like telemedicine (even a health service itself moves across frontiers), or helpful services that benefit from new medical information technologies. In real terms the factor that more than the others easily and frequently moves, is data, meaning all the documents that contain any kind of information on patient's condition and clinical details throughout the care path.

---

[2] Directive 2011/24/EU of the European Parliament and of the Council of 9 March 2011 on the application of patients' rights in cross-border healthcare. *Official Journal of the European Union*, 2011; L88: 45–46.

12.1.2 Patient Mobility: By Choice or By Necessity?

No unique underpinning stimulus is the leverage that brings patients to travel important distances for diagnosis and healthcare. One of the most significant incentives is the deficiency (or even the absence) of expertise and competences at national level or the impossibility to receive timely healthcare, inducing dissatisfaction and frustration in patients. Flaking this condition, there are categories of people that decide to travel to a foreign country looking for a high-quality healthcare or very specialized treatments not available in small member states. But many other factors are active elements of the mobility process. As mentioned, the peculiarity of living in cross-border regions is a relative common reason. Likewise, for citizens that share languages or cultural habits, it is easier to move to another country, or even people on vacations or temporary visits need access to healthcare services [1]. The situation is similar for long-term visitors from a European country to another or citizens from a European country who retire in a different member state and prefer to take advantages of its healthcare system. Another incentive behind patient mobility is the policy of particular countries for specific pathological area, such as for orphan diseases or for defined political measures.

12.1.3 Telemedicine

The roots of telemedicine lie in the aerospace history during the early 1960s by the need to monitor astronauts, like Yuri Gagarin, during space flights: a truly cross-border approach.

Since then, the field has been improved and implemented by contributions of innovation on information and communication technologies (ICTs), and nowadays telemedicine is recognized as one of the most important eHealth instruments.

Telemedicine, sometimes referred to as telehealth, is defined as "the delivery of health care services, where distance is a critical factor, by all health care professionals using ICTs for the exchange of valid information for diagnosis, treatment and prevention of disease and injuries, research and evaluation, and for the continuing education of health care providers, all in the interests of advancing the health of individuals and their communities" [2].

As a matter of fact, telehealth, connecting caregivers and patients in different locations, overcomes geographical barriers to provide various clinical supports.

The peculiarities of telecare are accessibility, efficiency, quality, and cost-effectiveness, just to mention the most important, and these are keys which facilitate patient diagnosis and clinical management among European member states.

12.1.4 Continuity of Care

"Continuity of care" is a complex term that includes several points of view and concerns many aspects. People frequently experience it as a protracted caring relation between patients and medical doctors, nurses, etc. and perceive the continuity as the integration and coordination of provided services [3]. On the other hand, for providers, a guarantee of a continuity of care brings a different connotation that implies the degree of coordination between specialists and teamworking, the quality of care, and its delivery over time.

In literature, the meaning is the extension of care beyond single procedures or specific episodes of disease, involving delivery of service by various providers, creating a consistent and rational care plan (continuum of care). Haggerty et al. in 2003 defined continuity of care as follows: "series of health care services is experienced as connected and coherent and is consistent with a patient's health needs and personal circumstances" [4].

Three main types of continuity of care have been individuated:

(a) Informational, as a transversal documented flow of information on single events and different providers able to overcome language and ICT difficulties
(b) Management continuity, intending a care based on common protocols and plans, timely delivered
(c) Relational continuum, which involves past, contemporary, and also future care

These three aspects of continuity of care are even more important across borders: healthcare does not include only different providers, but also the movement of a patient from a European healthcare system to another.

More than any other, the context of chronic rare conditions and aging-related diseases can be afflicted by discontinuity of medical records, fragmented care pathway, and language barriers [4–6], making the role of a registry even more significant.

12.1.5 Cross-Border Collaborations: ERN

Europe is working actively to foster healthcare and cooperation, not only providing the aforementioned directives on cross-border medicine, but also stimulating the creation of *transfrontalier* collaboration. First of all, European reference networks (ERNs) are encouraged by the EU Committee of Experts on Rare Diseases also to define recommendations for quality criteria for a coordinated sharing of expertise and resources on orphan disease scenario [7].

The goal of an ERN is the improvement of the overall quality and management of care at the European level, in a cluster of orphan diseases with similar needs, achieved by complementing, supporting, and providing added value to the existing services and expertise at the national level.

Such networking synergy is accomplished among centers of excellence. It aims at addressing diagnosis, epidemiology, prevention, etiology, and treatment and wants to produce standards of care, best-practice protocols, and healthcare plans for patient management as well as to improve research through collection and harmonization of information on rare disease patients. All these purposes are achieved by sharing the experience on disease registries and biospecimen biobanking and on trainings for patients and health professionals and through exchanging resources or supporting the creation and development of patient organization networks.

ERNs are the networking instruments identified by the European Community to improve care for European citizens.

12.2 Think Rare

As previously anticipated, rare diseases require particular attention, since rare disease patients frequently undergo late diagnosis and inadequate care. In the European Union, rare diseases are conditions with prevalence below 0.05 %. The European Commission on public health defines rare diseases as "life-threatening or chronically debilitating diseases which are of such low prevalence that special combined efforts are needed to address them." The Rare Disease Act of 2002 and the US Orphan Drug Act define a rare disease or condition as one that " (a) affects less than 200,000 persons in the United States, or (b) affects more than 200,000 in the United States and for which there is no reasonable expectation that the cost of developing and making available in the United States a drug for such disease or condition will be recovered from sales in the United States of such drug" [8]. Doing the math, this makes roughly 0.07 % of the US population.

Rare diseases might be wrongly considered to have little numeric impact. However, so far, 6 to 7000 distinct orphan diseases have been identified, 80 % of which are caused by 1 (or more) alteration on 1 (or more) gene among all different genes already identified. More or less 30 million people in the European Union are estimated to be affected by rare conditions (6–8 % of the population). Such vast numbers present key problems for healthcare and treatments and for research: the amount of available data is very limited and the range of required information types is enormous. In addition, more or less 75 % of rare diseases affects kids, and 30 % of them will die before the age of 5 [9].

The diagnosis sometimes (if not even frequently) requires several years, and treatments, if available, are dispensed when the disease has already caused impairments in patients, in terms of signs and symptoms and quality of life. Most rare diseases are currently not curable, primarily due to the lack of a deep understanding of the underlying disease mechanisms [10].

The peculiarities of orphan diseases, limited number of patients, and scarcity of relevant information, single them out as a specific scenario, and the management of these patients requires early identification and updated research information in order to perform suitable healthcare, proper treatment, and rapid diagnosis and assistance. Orphan diseases are defined by their distribution in local or global population. The rarity of the disease makes it crucial that information is shared by the medical community, otherwise the lack of knowledge, the gaps in clinical profiling, the insufficiency of consensus guidelines, and the absence of therapies can transform diagnosis and management in an odyssey both for patients and for medical doctors.

12.2.1 Osteochondrodysplasias

Skeletal dysplasias are a clinically and genetically heterogeneous group of rare disorders of the bone and/or cartilage, characterized by anomalies that determine defects in the growth, development, and maintenance of the human skeleton [11]. This group includes more than 430 diseases caused by mutations on 364 individuated gene(s); all the conditions are classified into three main subgroups – osteodysplasias, chondrodysplasias, and dysostoses – depending on alterations of bone density, cartilaginous development, and bone malformation, but diagnostic boundaries are frequently blurred. To this end, and to better classify osteochondrodysplasias, a few months ago, Bonafè et al. defined 42 main disease clusters according to clinical presentation, radiological features, and molecular characteristics [12]; the rarity of these conditions determines a limited availability of information on the current clinical procedures and the involvement of clinical, etiologic, and pathogenetic research, and planning of clinical studies is hindered. In other words, low prevalence of skeletal dysplasias determines minor knowledge and difficulties in application of the information in the clinical practice.

As for all orphan diseases, patients suffering from skeletal dysplasias are strongly disadvantaged, since the low prevalence of their conditions causes the absence of referral centers which could offer diagnosis, clinical treatments, and follow-up; this situation leads patients to be often not timely diagnosed and not adequately treated [13]. These diverse clusters of disorders necessitate an ad hoc management that comprises not only medical problems but also psychological and social difficulties.

12.3   The Power of a Patient Registry

Many definitions are available for patient registry. The US Agency for Healthcare Research and Quality define a registry as "an organized system that uses observational study methods to collect uniform data (clinical and other) to evaluate specified outcomes for a population defined by a particular disease, condition, or exposure, and that serves one or more predetermined scientific, clinical or policy purposes," and in 1974 WHO described it as "a file of documents containing uniform information about individual persons, collected in a systematic and comprehensive way, in order to serve a predetermined scientific, clinical or policy purpose" [14]. Many other descriptions can be found internationally, but all of them share a few main concepts: (a) the realization of an organized system, (b) denoted by uniformity of data, (c) related to a specific disease or precise group of patients, (d) and finalized to explicit purposes.

More in details, a patient registry is a powerful tool composed of interconnected elements that work jointly in order to create an organized collection of information. The word "registry" is composed of two related connotations, the act of register and the entry in a repository and, effectively, both meanings are involved in a patient registry. The items collected, like clinical data, laboratory test results, medical history, and so on, are primary to the scope, but all of them are connoted by consistent uniformity both in the nuance of data type composition and in structuring of data themselves.

The patient registry, as the name suggests, comprises by nature only information related to a particular group of persons, mainly patients that share a common element. Depending on the focus, the Parent JA in 2015 [15] has individuated three macrogroups:

1. Product registry: this instrument aims at collecting information on patient exposed to a healthcare product meaning pharmaceutical therapy, biomedical device, diagnostic tool, and so on. The exposure may be single like a single-dose drug or prolonged (i.e., chronic usage of a therapy).
2. Health service registry: this type of registry is focused on gathering data on exposure to a specific healthcare product or procedure. Examples of topics are patients who underwent a particular surgery or a person admitted to the hospital for a specific diagnosis.
3. Disease/condition registry: this tool applies a particular disease or condition as the inclusion criterion. The participants of this macrogroup are registry-enrolling patients affected by a lifelong disease (i.e., rare diseases) or persons suffering from a condition for a limited period of time.

Whatever the preferred type of patient registry, a registry must be designed to accomplish specific finalities and established with respect to final defined purposes: to perform epidemiological studies or investigations on natural history (in terms of management, characteristics, and outcomes), to determine cost-effective analyses or clinical efficiency evaluation, and also to monitor safety or to measure quality; in fact in the large amount of cases, a registry has multiple aims.

12.4 The Patient Registry as a Tool for Cross-Border Healthcare

To achieve a complete and meaningful overview of persons affected by hereditary rare diseases, to guarantee rare skeletal dysplasia patients to be adequately followed, and to support diagnosis of orphan patients (a process that may require several years), designing and running a registry is the solution, especially in the light of Directive 2011/24/EU.

Comprehending clinical phenotypes through their corresponding genotypes is fundamental to unveil inherited mutations that could lead to pathological processes and syndromes. But linking genetic alterations and clinical evidences, in diseases that affect a small percentage of the population, is obviously problematic due to, as mentioned, the scarcity of resources, the scattering of data, and the knowledge fragmentation. As a matter of fact, orphan diseases impose data merge from dispersed sources: usually, a single research center lacks sufficient resources to conduct meaningful research, and data must be collected and shared by different partners (hospitals, research centers, and other facilities) in order to individuate best clinical procedures, to update treatments, and to provide an accurate diagnosis. Moreover, clinical, genomic, and imaging data and pedigree combination is necessary to create a comprehensive disease view, to avoid redundant instances, and to solve the long-standing problem of incomplete information. The patient registry solves the need of an improved instrument to speed up diagnosis and to facilitate management and treatment across borders.

12.4.1 An Example of Patient Registry Platform: GePhCARD

The Medical Genetic Department of Rizzoli Orthopaedic Institute in collaboration with a local software house, Nier IT Solution (NSI), has designed a digital platform, named genotype-phenotype correlation, analyses, and research database (GePhCARD), that focuses on combining mutational screening and phenotypic outcomes to investigate disease pathophysiology. The software is concretely *transfrontalier*, since it is Web accessible by any Internet browser (intranet/Internet connection), and it has been realized with logical and intuitive interfaces for the end user.

GePhCARD is designed as a multi-client system, allowing secure storage, retrieval, and rationalization of data from disperse locations. The platform enables on-demand data mining and integration of new and/or existing services and applications and it is easily achieved. Moreover, it complies with the current state-of-the-art standards in medical informatics, like Health Level Seven (HL7) and Digital Imaging and Communications in Medicine (DICOM), to ensure dialogue openness, flexibility, and extendibility [16–18]. Since the end users of the platform are not IT specialists, the user interface experience was designed in a straightforward and intuitive way.

Frequently, the systems used to collect data are paper based or spreadsheets flanked by (paper) medical reports, a common scenario of several groups researching on rare diseases. Via GePhCARD it is possible to dematerialize all paper-based documents and improve information collected.

A separate information relative to the clinic data, to the samples and specimens, and, above all, to the genetic data as a patient registry for genotype-phenotype correlation has been reported on this platform. As mentioned before, GePhCARD has been realized following a modularity principle, allowing clinical and genetic domain extensibility (i.e., new methods for molecular screening data, including the storage of documents in a customizable folder structure system (documental domain extensibility).

The platform in addition to providing legal security and over time stability of data, can manage different log-ins and roles by a designed tool for multilevel data access, thereby protecting the patient. The multilevel access profile system takes care of data legal protection using an authentication system based on a username and password; the idea was the creation of different roles with different accessibility skills (to read, to write, to modify previous inserted data). The patient data accessibility is based on a role-based access control (RBAC) system that provides users from different organizations with customized access rights to patients' information according to the user profile or role. By this GePhCARD keeps traceability (user, organization, and date) of all patient's creation and modification, visualizing them on each patient data page. Users' roles are predefined and assigned during the user creation, and the RBAC controller servlet is responsible to define user rights for each form, panel inside a form, toolbar, and menu bar.

Another striking improvement is the data sharing via Internet connection and the consequent opportunity of a constant update of data and the real-time access from multiple locations (ambulatory, day clinic, molecular lab, etc.), a perfect solution for a cross-border tool. This interoperability is supported by common standard protocol HL7, recognized as the standard for healthcare data exchange; accordingly the upload/retrieve of family history data is realized according to HL7 v2/v3 Family History standards.

12.4.2 GePhCARD Infrastructure

GePhCARD is designed and developed according to the service-oriented architecture (SOA) principles; collecting data modules (disease, technique, etc.) have been individuated in advance and designed as services (Web services) and then plugged into the overall architecture to ensure the interoperability and cooperation among the different modules [19]. It consists of the following software components:

- A relational database to store clinical, genomic, and genealogic data of patients
- A relational database to store and index digital documents (mainly DICOM images produced by PACS systems of healthcare organizations)
- A document management system based on Alfresco framework to manage any kind of documents collected for each patient [20]
- A Web application to provide users with a common graphical user interface (GUI)

In the main Java Web application, designed and built according to J2EE standards, 20 is responsible for providing end users with a large set of GUIs to manage all the data of patients.

12.4.3 The Achieved Results

This type of sharing has allowed us to create three patient registries, (a) registry of hereditary multiple exostoses (REM), (b) osteogenesis imperfecta registry (ROI), and (c) registry of Ehler-Danlos syndrome (RED), and enabled us to collect very large numbers of rare patients, achieving a dataset of more than 1300 patients affected by exostoses (the largest dataset worldwide), about 650 patients affected by osteogenesis imperfecta, and 350 patients suffering from Ehler-Danlos syndrome; however, these numbers continue to grow.

It should also be pointed out that the use of combo box, in addition to speed up the collection of information, results in a reduction of typing errors (typos), an advantage which is reflected greatly in the quality of the data. In fact all modules and sections are provided, when possible, with fixed drop-down list (easily upgradeable by the administrator) for easier and faster field filling in order to complete all data sections more quickly.

Moreover, this platform allows users to perform searches on structured data, to select case studies and to export them on spreadsheets for further investigations or analyses with statistical and predictive software. GePhCARD exporting tool was also applied for selection and extraction of specific sub-cohorts of patients, in order to explain interindividual variability in specific clinical characteristics or for selection of unrelated patients undergoing genetic and orthopedic visit for validation of a new diagnostic protocol.

Safety and security is pursued through a data loss prevention plan that implies a scheduled backup (on an external memory disk) every 24 h, resulting in a continuous data protection. The result files are very lightweight, despite the fact that entire dataset includes a huge amount of patients accompanied by clinical, genetic, and genealogical data.

In conclusion, this platform for patient registry is a powerful instrument to study hereditary diseases, both Mendelian and multifactorial, enabling physicians to evaluate diseases with a patient centric approach, and helps researchers for *transfrontalier* studies planning.

12.5   Personal Considerations

The common way of storage for clinical and genetic data is often chaotic and sometimes inconvenient (sometimes even unsafe), especially when dealing with rare disease scenario. We created a patient registry platform for improving patient management and, at the same time, for helping researchers for analyses on specific cohort of patients. An essential issue is the data merge from different institutions and cross-borders to perform analyses that could reach statistical significance. GePhCARD fulfills these needs contributing to collection, storage, management, integration, and analysis of the phenotype and genotype data from different European sources and allowing patient follow-up with a better accuracy.

GePhCARD provides users the chance to survey disease progression and to evaluate targets for a focused clinical research. Accessibility and high-quality representation is key to a productive usage of the system. To increase the user friendliness, we have planned a multi-language engine and a multi-organization structure that make the software suitable for being utilized by dispersed clinical and research organizations. Moreover, the interface for the World Wide Web has been developed to provide an easy condition to accumulate data on many scales, from genomic to clinical, driving to the formation of a backbone for orphan pathologies considered. While none of the data collected are unique when considered alone, their combination is unique and may represent an important contribution to disease comprehension.

To conclude, the introduction of GePhCARD has led to a larger and better delineated, both clinically and genetically, dataset resulting in a more accurate patient follow-up. This allows a safer and more secure protection of data form the patient (privacy) and the researcher (stability over time) perspective. In addition, the dataset will be more up-to-date, with less typo and will be easily exportable to promote specific investigations or enquiries.

We are day by day acquiring knowledge on this transversal scenario that covers biomedical and scientific problems but also faces many legal, ICT, and ethical issues that support both diagnosis and research, implementing our platform and the three patient registries REM, ROI, and RED leaning on it.

Cross-border medicine, continuity of care, and ERN need a pooling of information, in particular in diagnosis and care of rare disease scenario that requires very specialized knowledge for comprehension of pathology and patient management. This pathology-oriented IT instrument can provide an organized pooling of patient information; a structured description of clinical signs, genetic results, and familiar data; and the opportunity to perform statistics. Thanks to all these peculiarities, the patient registry platform brings healthcare professionals to a complete overview of disease, to an individuation of sub-cohort of patients with specific manifestations (that are responsive, or not, to a determined treatment), to an identification of disease-causative pathways, etc. As a result, a disease registry can help doctors in providing high-quality and cost-effective healthcare.

References

1. Rosenmoller M, McKee M, Baeten R (eds) (2006) Patient Mobility in the European Union: Learning from Experience. European Observatory on Health Systems and Policies, Copenhagen
2. WHO (1998) A health telematics policy in support of WHO's Health-For-All strategy for global health development: report of the WHO group consultation on health telematics, Geneva, 11–16 Dec 1997. World Health Organization, Geneva
3. Gulliford M, Naithani S, Morgan M (2006) What is 'continuity of care'? J Health Serv Res Policy 11(4):248–250
4. Haggerty JL, Reid RJ, Freeman GK, Starfield BH, Adair CE, Rachael MK (2003) Continuity of care: a multidisciplinary review. BMJ 327(7425):1219–1221. doi:10.1136/bmj
5. Legido-Quigley H, Glinos IA, Baeten R, McKee M, Busse R (2012) Analysing arrangements for cross-border mobility of patients in the European Union: a proposal for a framework. Health Policy 108:27–36
6. Panteli D, Wagner C, Verheyen F, Busse R (2015) Know before you go': information-seeking behaviour of German patients receiving health services abroad in light of the provisions of Directive 2011/24/EU. J Health Serv Res Policy 20(3):154–161. doi:10.1177/1355819615580003, Epub 2015 Apr 20
7. Ségolène A, Charlotte R (2014) The European Union Committee of Experts on Rare Diseases: three productive years at the service of the rare disease community. Orphanet J Rare Dis 9:30. doi:10.1186/1750-1172-9-30
8. Orphan Drug Act. U.S. Food and Drug Administration http://www.fda.gov/regulatoryinformation/legislation/federalfooddrugandcosmeticactfdcact/significantamendmentstothefdcact/orphandrugact/default.htm
9. Rare Disease UK. National alliance for people with rare diseases. Available at: http://www.raredisease.org.uk/

10. Office of the Secretary, DoD (2010) TRICARE; rare diseases definition. Fed Regist 75(151):47458
11. Spranger J, Brill P, Poznanski A (2002) Bone dysplasias. An Atlas of genetic disorders of skeletal development, 2nd edn. Oxford University Press, New York
12. Luisa Bonafe, Valerie Cormier-Daire, Christine Hall, Ralph Lachman, Geert Mortier, Stefan Mundlos, Gen Nishimura, Luca Sangiorgi, Ravi Savarirayan, David Sillence, Jurgen Spranger, Andrea Superti-Furga, Matthew Warman, and Sheila (2015) Unger nosology and classification of genetic skeletal disorders. revision. AJMG 2015 Sep 23. doi: 10.1002/ajmg.a.37365
13. Savariryan R, Rimoin DL (2002) The skeletal dysplasias. Best Pract Res Clin Endocrinol Metab 16(3):547–560
14. Gliklich RE, Dreyer NA (2010) Registries for evaluating patient outcomes: a user's guide, 2nd edn. Agency for Healthcare Research and Quality, Rockville, AHRQ Publication No.10-EHC049
15. Metka Zaletel, Marcel Kralj eds (2015) Methodological guidelines and recommendations for efficient and rational governance of patient registries. Oct.
16. Dolin RH, Alschuler L, Boyer S, Beebe C, Behlen FM, Byron PV et al (2006) HL7 clinical document architecture, release 2. J Am Med Inform Assoc 13(1):30–39
17. Health Level 7. http://www.hl7.org/
18. Cong Y, Zhihong Y (2009) XML-based DICOM data format. J Digit Imaging 23–2:192–202
19. Douglas KB (2003) Web services and service-oriented architectures: the savvy manager's guide. Morgan Kaufmann Publishers, San Francisco
20. Open Source Document Management System by Alfresco. http://www.alfresco.com/products/document-management/

Cross-Border Experiences in Health IT: What Are the Requests for the Medical Record? Opportunities and Emerging Issues

13

Dorjan Marušič, Valentina Prevolnik Rupel, and Peter Mihelj

13.1 Introduction

The EU directive on cross-border healthcare was passed in 2011. The directive grants a fundamental right to purchase healthcare services across the European Economic Area (EEA) for all EEA citizens and the right to apply for reimbursement from their home system. Cross-border collaboration offers the potential to improve the performance of health systems at local, regional and national level, improving access and sharing experiences. However, there are many challenges to use and successfully implement offered and available potentials. Cross-border collaboration is complicated because collaborating partners are bound by the rules of their health systems. As these rarely coincide, partners need permissions from competent authorities or to invent solutions. Moreover, stakeholders react to domestic incentives and constraints, even when these are played out locally.

There are many challenges in cross-border healthcare that are connected to Information technology (IT), and we will try to expose some of them and understate them by using existing and practical examples from European-level projects and cooperation in healthcare in border region between Slovenia and Italy. As IT solutions are mostly used within externally financed projects and are not widely applicable, the chapter will end by presenting an innovative solution called healthcare portal platforms. These are innovative Information communication technology (ICT) solutions that establish a collaborative system for medical experts and patients to actively participate in the healthcare process. Their role exceeds the standard practice as they do not serve just for the transfer of the data but are left contextually

D. Marušič (✉) • P. Mihelj
Tetras d.o.o., Koper, Slovenia
e-mail: dorjan.marusic@gmail.com

V.P. Rupel
Institute for Economic Research, Ljubljana, Slovenia
e-mail: dorjan.marusic@gmail.com

© Springer International Publishing Switzerland 2017
G. Rinaldi (ed.), *New Perspectives in Medical Records*, TELe-Health,
DOI 10.1007/978-3-319-28661-7_13

empty if the patients and medical staff are not involved in it in real time. Their involvement depends on the development of clear telemedicine clinical pathways that will assure trust and interest on all sides and consequently help stimulate collaboration between patients and medical workers in a standardised and controlled environment.

13.2   Directive on Cross-Border Healthcare

The concept of cross-border cooperation in health is enshrined in article 168 of the Treaty on the Functioning of the European Union (TFEU). European Union policy in the field of health is aimed at complementing and supporting national health policies, encouraging cooperation between member states (MS) and promoting coordination between their programmes. The general mandate contained in the Treaty has been spelled out in Directive 2011/24/EU on the application of patients' rights in cross-border healthcare, which seeks to establish rules to facilitate access to safe and high-quality cross-border healthcare and ensure patient mobility in the Union, as well as promoting cooperation in healthcare between MS.

The legal mandate established by the public health article 168 of the TFEU explicitly recognises the potential added value for patients of cross-border collaboration, in particular "to improve the complementarity of health services". To this end, the commission may take "any useful initiative" that will help to coordinate MS' policies and programmes. In addition to concluding cross-border agreements, other suggested instruments are joint planning; mutual recognition or adaptation of procedures, standards, guidelines or indicators; interoperability of respective national ICT systems; practical mechanisms to ensure continuity of care or practical facilitating of cross-border provision of healthcare by health professionals on a temporary or occasional basis; exchange of best practice; and periodic monitoring and evaluation. It should be noted that all these possible initiatives are to be situated within forms of non-legislative cooperation and exchange between member states.

The Directive on cross-border care has been regarded by many as a major achievement of the policy of "patient empowerment", promoted by the EU, granting EU citizens the right to access healthcare services in another MS. The Directive aims to promote cooperation on healthcare between MS. The main risks to health and safety that may arise during cross-border care involve the management of complications requiring follow-up care, discontinuity of care caused by failure to coordinate medical documentation and incomplete information to permit informed decision-making. For these reasons, formal actions are needed to ensure access to safe and high-quality cross-border healthcare and patient mobility within the European Union (EU). These should, first, establish that there are mechanisms within each MS assuring that the care provided is of high quality, with specific additional measures to address issues arising when patients cross borders to obtain care, as well as those that deal with their needs for aftercare following their return.

Currently, there are many examples within the EU of bilateral agreements between MS or their health agencies or insurance companies that enable access to health services in another MS, often negotiated with little or no reference to EU law. There is much that can be learned from these examples, such as measures taken in regions with high tourist inflows, both during summer and winter seasons, that have demonstrated the feasibility of reorganising their healthcare systems to respond. There is also considerable accumulated experience in offering health services through multilateral agreements for people living abroad (pensioners, those temporarily staying in other country, etc.). The European Health Insurance Card is just one manifestation of this developments.

Cross-border collaboration offers the potential to improve the performance of health systems at local, regional and national level, improving access and sharing experiences. In Europe that allows for the free mobility of patients, health professionals, medical devices and pharmaceuticals, performance improvements must not end at national borders. The internal market was created to raise Europe's economic performance by merging national labour, commodity, service and capital markets. It would be a bitter irony if patients, professionals, providers and financing institutions could not benefit from these opportunities.

However, there are other issues to be considered. Patient mobility also means that providers in one member state may, in some circumstances, effectively be in competition with providers in other one, where competition arises from patient choice (or by someone acting on behalf of the patient). Even if patients do not utilise the possibility for cross-border care, the mere existence of this option may, at least in theory, encourage care providers to become more responsive to patient needs. For example, if all providers in an MS improve their quality in a similar way, an impact on quality would be observed. However, as long as the relative qualities remain unchanged, patients have no reason to move more than before [17]. Thus, mobility of patients may impact on quality, but the absence of mobility does not necessarily imply that there is no impact from the potential to move.

13.3   Challenges of Cross-Border IT

Cross-border patient mobility [15] is the most commonly used expression within the EU to describe a social phenomenon that involves people crossing a border to receive healthcare.

Advances in electronic communications have enabled patients in one member state to be diagnosed and treated by health professionals in another member state by means of telemedicine. The biggest systematic review in the area of cross-border healthcare was conducted that included 94 papers on the use of telemedicine to deliver cross-border healthcare and identify the factors that hinder or support its implementation [15]. They involved 76 countries worldwide, most involving collaborations between high- and low- and middle-income countries. Most described services delivered a combination of types of telemedicine but specialties most represented were tele-pathology, telesurgery, emergency and trauma telemedicine and tele-radiology. Most link health professionals, with only a few linking professionals directly to patients. A main driver for the development of cross-border telemedicine is the need to improve access to specialist services in low- and middle-income countries and in underserved rural areas in high-income countries. Factors that hinder or support implementation are clustered into four main themes: (1) legal factors, (2) sustainability factors, (3) cultural factors and (4) contextual factors.

Legal factors in the provision of cross-border healthcare are important if we want to ensure safety and quality of healthcare services. In the field of informatisation, legal factors refer to movement of patient data across borders – such movement requires patients' informed consent to data sharing and storage. It is obvious that data safety and protection are not at the same levels across countries, so such concerns are specially relevant in the countries where legal clarity regarding data protection and storage is lacking at national level [14].

The financial sustainability of telemedicine still remains a critical issue, regardless of the rapid decline in the cost of technology over the last few years: due to drop in costs of the technology, the sustainability issue does not refer to start-up costs but to costs for technical maintenance; in any case, these are outweighed by personnel and management costs [14]. A much bigger issue than financial sustainability is the acceptance of technology-based solution that would promote remote healthcare services by staff members. As technological solutions are not yet integrated into national health systems in terms of reimbursement, the staff members are only partially attracted to them (mostly in the pilots or externally financed projects).

It is inevitable that cross-border healthcare will also be tackled with different languages, cultural differences arising from different working methods, patterns of communication and perception of privacy.

All these factors were found in various studies that studied healthcare in connection to information technology use across border. A qualitative study of a teleradiology clinic in Barcelona, offering services to hospitals in a range of European countries, was undertaken to identify the challenges faced in providing such a service [9]. It identified the need for a clear legal framework, especially in relation to areas such as redress and liability and comparability of clinical governance arrangements. For example, patients in Sweden benefit from a no-fault compensation scheme when treated by domestic providers, but this does not extend to providers established abroad. In other areas there is a European legal framework, such as data transfer, but one member state, the UK, insisted on additional, highly complex provisions [9]. These studies provide a basis for further legal clarification to ensure quality and safety [13].

Challenges in delivering telemedicine services across borders, for example, stirred the confusion about whether the health professionals involved must be licensed in all countries where patients are being treated [15]. Reproductive care is one of the most common reasons why people cross borders for healthcare [12]. In this area legal challenges are connected to issues of citizenship. One example can be shown in a case of initiative to support Italian women giving birth in Slovenia. Italian women living in border regions with Slovenia could use Slovenian hospital, as it is their closest health facility, to give birth. However, initiative was not too successful as Italian women asked for official confirmation from Italian municipalities that their children were born in Italy; also hospital in Slovenia wanted a guarantee that Italy will pay the costs. Always existent and challenging are issues regarding data summaries and patient registries. The results of different projects have identified privacy issues and data sensitivity issues within national legislation.

When providing cross-border care, informatisation and digitalisation even further gain on importance as more data is moved across the borders with patients. The first challenge is connected to the level of digitalisation. There are big differences in levels of digitalisation among member states. Different levels of healthcare systems, especially regarding the infrastructure, present one of the main obstacles in the cross-border project implementation. Smaller hospitals do not provide a complete range of services and cannot afford to purchase or maintain high-tech systems – all these issues could and should be tackled through the reorganisation of the provider network at the national level.

Besides digitalisation, interoperability of information systems and e-health technologies is crucial in the process of providing quality and safe healthcare. Standardisation of telemedicine is not a regulated area and many different, often conflicting standards or different versions and implementations of the same standard are used. Consequently, there is a big problem in the interoperability of information systems and e-health technologies. Integration of information systems for communication and exchange of data with other systems on the basis of standardised protocols and interfaces are tough issues. Interoperability is a wider concept of integration – upgrade of communication means in actual interaction to increase efficiency and reduce costs. It might be that the open source approach can be a promise.

In spite of stating information technology issues as challenges, it is important to stress that technology per se cannot be an obstacle. Technology is used in all other sectors, and there are successful international IT projects in almost all industries. Healthcare remains one of the last nonintegrated sectors. Standards, as well, are not a problem as standards are defined in medicine informatics (HL7 and IHE) that define interoperability and exchange of data, security, terminology dictionaries and protocols for authorisation, identification and authentication of patients. Moreover there are several proofs of concepts where these standards and regulations were already used and implemented, for example, epSOS project [8] that covered more than 45 members from 22 EU member states and three non-EU member states. epSOS aimed to design, build and evaluate a service infrastructure that demonstrates cross-border interoperability among electronic health record (EHR) systems in Europe. Nevertheless, cross-border IT projects in healthcare are in a very early stage and do not evolve after EU funding for piloting stops. Creation of competition across borders [10] can have unintended negative consequences for both communication between providers and access to care. Cross-border collaborations can face multiple logistical barriers, and developing solutions requires the commitment of many actors. Attention to communication between providers in the form of discharge summaries and assigned contact persons is important for ensuring continuity of care.

The main challenge remains implementation of standards in whole EU members and *enforcement of legislations and governances in healthcare*. Additionally, it is very important to establish *quality measurements and quality protocols that will enable seamless healthcare to all European citizens in all EU countries*. Quality of care [10] issues are likely to arise when cross-border care falls outside of such arrangements. Measures to ensure quality of care for all patients receiving care across borders include strengthening implementation of clinical guidelines, standardisation of discharge summary content, appropriate regulation of professional standards, optimal use of technologies such as telemedicine and e-health records and management of language barriers through interpreters and language training for health professionals. Such measures are likely to have positive impacts on quality of care for patients receiving care in their home country as well as those who travel abroad.

13.4 Examples of Cross-Border Cooperation/Collaboration in Italy and Slovenia

Cross-border collaboration offers scope to exchange best practices and test them in relevant environments, supports harmonisation of measures to ensure quality of care and provides a basis for effective legislation.

IntegrAid (Integrated Approach to Improve Emergency Medical Assistance in Cross-Border) aimed to ensure optimal care of patients at risk living in the cross-border area through harmonisation of the emergency medical services, professional medical qualification, use of tele-consultations and improvement of the logistics system.

E-health in the border region aimed to increase the quality of life through the coordinated development of health and social systems using information and communication technology. A common network was created using bilingual digitised cross-border clinical records. This seeks to facilitate mobility and traceability of patients and ensure tele-counselling and professional training. The E-surgerynet project (surgical network in the border region) proposed the creation of excellence network of cross-border surgery in order to implement clinical, organisational and management models and dissemination of standard protocols. A common technology platform will enable specialist consultations live and on-demand sessions to create a video library and a surgical e-learning area dedicated to vocational training. In the e-CardioNet (Network Cardiology in the border region), new administrative practices were introduced, as well as innovative clinical models in the treatment of heart failure, emergency surgery and a more multidisciplinary approach to rehabilitation and secondary prevention. The project creates a network to ensure the patient care in emergency angioplasty and cardiac surgery in hospitals close to the border and apply new protocols for the prevention and treatment of heart failure and an access to online services and archives for cardiologists and health professionals.

Sanicademia [16], officially known as the International Academy for Health Professionals (EEIG), is a euroregional academy for health professionals of the Italian Regions of Friuli-Venezia Giulia and the Veneto and the Austrian Land, Carinthia. The school caters to the training needs of medical doctors, nurses and health workers at large. It is supported at the highest political levels in the three regions. The academy has taken advantage of a number of European structural funds within the framework of an Interreg IVA-supported project "cross-border collaboration in patient care" between Austria and Italy. The Academy's main goal is to provide a systematic exchange of information, experiences and expertise between regional healthcare systems and to provide a sort of permanent public health training "campus" which extends across borders. Up to now, professional training credits granted to doctors and nurses have been recognised only in their own countries; therefore, Sanicademia has made it one of its priorities to pull down these "administrative barriers" by exploring ways of creating qualifications which are recognised across borders. A number of local health units in the Northeast regions of Italy, in Carinthia and in Slovenia are actively enrolling their staff in Sanicademia as part of their skills improvement programmes.

Trans2care (T2C) [11] was a project to promote knowledge dissemination and technology transfer, favouring innovative practices and products for disease prevention, early diagnosis, personalised therapies, safety monitoring of the environment and the food chain between Slovenia and Italy. T2C was aimed at creating an international network operating in a range of scientific fields, seeking to develop new products and services for the improvement of the health system.

13.5   Healthcare Platform

Healthcare portal platforms are innovative ICT solutions that establish a collaborative system for medical experts and patients to actively participate in the healthcare process. They help to stimulate collaboration between patients and medical workers in a standardised and controlled environment. Health information technology [3] with real-time interactions can enhance the effects of chronic disease management, particularly when used in conjunction with behaviour change programmes.

Portal platform addresses two important factors which are changing the organisation of healthcare sector and roles of patients and doctors in the healing process. First challenge represents a new generation of medical professionals which are recognising the potential clinical benefits of having the whole patient record at their fingertips. With [1] Electronic Health Records, information is available whenever and wherever it is needed. As a new generation of medical professionals will gain seniority in healthcare practices, demand and acceptance will sharply increase. The second factor is active participation of patients in the healing process. Patient engagement [2] is an increasingly important component of strategies to reform healthcare. Patients want to be active in the healing process; they want to have access to their medical records and want to understand how healing process is planned, what are the next activities and what are triggers to start the next step in the healing process. Patient portals [4] can offer important benefits to patients and provider organisations. These technologies – particularly when integrated with an electronic health record (EHR) – have the potential to improve both quality and access to care through features that enable patients to communicate electronically and securely with their provider, access their medical records, schedule appointments, pay bills and refill prescriptions.

Portal platforms are new in healthcare and still in the early phase of development. There are not many studies covering healthcare portal platforms and also not many best practices and solutions. There are many misleads and wrong implementations of portals in healthcare. Moreover, portals in healthcare cannot be used in all situations and cannot cover all treatment procedures. Patient portals [5] seem to offer great potential for higher quality care, but it is unknown whether providers who offer the portals will be able to capitalise on the meaningful use stage 2 incentive due to lack of awareness of the patient portal service. Portals enable collaboration and at the same time require active, consistent and regular participations of all users. There are good examples of usage of healthcare portals for chronic patients and paediatric cases. Most users [6] fall into three groups – young parents, family members caring for elderly parents and patients with chronic illnesses. But these are early adopters of portals in medicine. There are still many opportunities for massive usage of using health portals.

An open area for healthcare portals is cross-border collaboration, migrations and tourist travelling. These groups urgently need support and access to their medical records and continuing healing process especially in case of chronic patients. This challenge was managed in the AdriHealthMob (AHM) project which is realised within the Priority 3 of the IPA Adriatic Cross-Border Cooperation Programme and responds to the need to strengthen and integrate the infrastructure networks, promoting the accessibility of health and care services. The project foresees the participation of 15 partners from the eight countries that constitute the Macro-Adriatic Region. One significant project result is delivery of an innovative portal platform than can support migrations of patients and collaboration of medical experts in the Adriatic and Ionian region.

Portal platform represents a first step to address new healthcare organisation initiatives and supports mobility of patients from different countries and regions in this case in AHM project. With portal platform it is possible to connect all medical institutions of AHM project from all participating countries: Albania, Bosnia and Herzegovina, Croatia, Greece, Italy, Montenegro, Slovenia and Serbia. Portal platform enables to collect and present data from different remote monitoring devices and to collect and present data from environmental monitoring devices and collaboration of medical experts. Medical experts are able to communicate with medical experts from AHM countries, open a second opinion case and create a medical summary in a CDA format. This portal, built on top of interoperable middleware, enables patients to monitor and record various physical parameters, acquired by standardised and certified medical protocols, including medical-grade devices. Portal platform is based on international standards in medicine informatics. Consequently, it is possible to integrate additional medical institutions and other partners from AHM project or external.

AHM portal platform is a light and an intuitive web platform. It enables cross-border reviewing of patient's personal data and its vital signs, enables analysing and managing of this data to better understand patient's condition, defines a diagnosis and makes better clinical decision for better patient care. Additionally it enables creation of medical summary and second opinion and spreads and stimulates collaboration between medical experts. AHM portal platform is an excellent foundation to upgrade and expand it with national and regional cross-border healthcare solutions. Portal platform enables exchange of data and interoperability, but lacks management of medical data and support for creation, management and maintenance of clinical pathways and algorithms. This is a next challenge that portal platform must achieve to start massive usage. Data [7] is inherently dumb. It does not do anything unless you know how to use it, how to act on it, because algorithms are where the real value lies. Algorithms define action. Clinical pathways require additional study and research between different countries, before the upgrade of portal platform. It is important to understand how care pathways are implemented in different countries, how they can be compared with one another and what needs to be done to make them compatible.

Conclusions

In the area of IT use in cross-border healthcare, there are a lot of opportunities. Although the Directive on cross-border healthcare has been around since 2011, the opportunities have not been exhausted in depth. While there have been many projects and pilot implementations of IT technology, we can claim that the major move from project-based collaboration to formal cross-border service provision with the use of IT has not yet happened. Although there are still lots of challenges before people will be indifferent between using care at home and care abroad, them being of legal, financial, contextual or cultural nature, none of them can be seen as paramount and could be solved in short term. Cross-border healthcare adds a new dimension of technology use for its strong emphasis on prevention of ill health before curative care. A whole paradigm shift is needed as current health systems are organised mainly to cure – successfulness of such a shift would contribute to the enhanced provision of cross-border services with higher use of IT solutions.

To achieve this goal, mechanisms need to be created to share best practice in areas such as medical records, prescriptions and e-health, to improve collaboration between those working in different health systems. Telemedicine can improve scheduling, patient satisfaction and compliance with treatment plans, increase reimbursements and more efficiently share information with other providers.

References

1. Levingston SA (2012) Opportunities in physician electronic health records: a road map for vendors. Bloomberg Government, New York
2. Hibbard JH, Greene J (2013) What the evidence shows about patient activation: better health outcomes and care experiences; fewer data on costs. Health Aff 2013(32):2207–2214
3. Cohen SB, Grote KD, Pietraszek WE, Laflamme F (2010) Increasing consumerism in healthcare trough intelligent information technology. Am J Manag Care 2010(16):SP37–SP43
4. Emont S (2011) Measuring the impact of Patient portals. California Healthcare Foundation. Available at: www.chcf.org. Accessed 30 Oct 2015)

5. Kruse CS, Bolton K, Kruse GF (2015) The effect of patient portals on quality outcomes and its implications to meaningful use: a systematic review. J Med Internet Res 17:2, Available at: http://www.jmir.org. Accessed 2 Nov 2015
6. Gardner E (2010) Will patients portal open the door to better care? Health Data Manag Mag 18:58
7. Sondergaard P (2015) It's not just about big data; it's what you do with it: welcome to the algorithmic economy. Gartner Symposium ITxpo 2015. Available at: http://www.gartner.com/newsroom/id/3142917. Accessed 2 Nov 2015
8. European Patients Smart Open Services (ePSOS) Available at: http://www.epsos.eu/home/project-members-beneficiaries.html. Accessed 2 Nov 2015
9. Legido-Quigley H, La Parra Casado D (2007) The health care needs of UK pensioners living in Spain: an agenda for research. Eurohealth 13:14–18
10. Footman K, Knai C, Baeten R, Glonti K, McKee M (2014) Cross-border health care in Europe. Available at: http://www.lse.ac.uk/LSEHealthAndSocialCare/pdf/Cross-border-health-care-in-Europe-Eng.pdf. Accessed on 30 Oct 2015
11. Transregional Network for Innovation and Technology Transfer to Improve Health Care (trans2care). Available at: http://www.trans2care.eu/Sections.aspx?section=452. Accessed 2 Nov 2015
12. Hudson N, Culley L, Blyth E et al (2011) Cross-border reproductive care: a review of the literature. Reprod Biomed 22(7):673–685
13. Glinos IA (2013) Hospitals and borders: seven case-studies on cross-border collaboration. EuroHealth Obs 19(4):21–23
14. Aaviksoo A, Kruus P (2013) Cross-border potential of telemedicine solutions. EuroHealth Obs 19(4):24–25
15. Saliba V, Legido-Quigley H, Hallik R, Aaviksoo A, Car J, Mckee M (2012) Telemedicine across borders: a systematic review of factors that hinder or support implementation. Int J Med Inform 81(12):793–809
16. Bertinato L, Canapero M (2009) Successful Cross-Border Education and Training: The Example of sanicademia. In: Polak, G. [Hg.]: Medicine & Health, Going International, Vienna, pg. 144–148
17. Hanefeld J, Lunt N, Simth RD, Horsfall DG (2015) Why do medical tourists travel to where they do? The role of networks in determining medical travel. Social science and Medicine 124:356–363

Innovative Tools and Data Sharing in Aged Care: Solutions and Perspectives

14

Ilir Qose

When the implementation of technology is evaluated, the social care component, and the role that innovation can play in this sector are often underestimated during the technology assesme. This chapter is based on the experience of Cooss Marche, an Italian non-profit social care provider, in piloting and utilizing existing innovative technology, improving and integrating the care process.

The concept of de-institutionalization differs from that of de-hospitalization; in relation to de-institutionalization, technological tools, usually non-medical devices, can be used to assist older adults to live well at home. These tools can be to coordinate and support services, and to organize personal and care information, communicating with all actors involved in the care process, in home monitoring, and in helpline systems. Under the pilot actions of the AdriHealthMob Project, innovative hardware and software, already on the market, are included in the personalized integrated care service packages made available to users in the Marche region in Italy.

14.1   Introduction

Cooss Marche is a social business based in Ancona, Italy. Created in 1979, it actually is a lead player in Care Sector Services at Italian Market, with 2,500 partners-employees. One of the specific features of Cooss Marche as a social care provider, is that, in 1993, it implemented a Research and Development Department that is focused on social needs research, innovation deployment, and European Union (EU)-funded project management.

In 2013, Cooss Marche was awarded the AdriHealthMob strategic project, under the Adriatic IPA Cbc program (Adriatic IPA (Instrument for Pre Accession Assistance) Cross Border Cooperation Programme), aiming at improving mobility

I. Qose
Cooperativa Sociale Cooss Marche Onlus Scpa, Ancona, Italy
e-mail: ilir.qose@gmail.com

© Springer International Publishing Switzerland 2017
G. Rinaldi (ed.), *New Perspectives in Medical Records*, TELe-Health,
DOI 10.1007/978-3-319-28661-7_14

in the health and care sector, both locally and in other countries involved in the project. One of the tasks under Cooss Marche coordination is demonstrating the role that innovation and information and communications technology (ICT) tools play in the improvement of the care sector; in particular, how these innovative tools can be introduced in the care process, reducing unnecessary immobility and increasing rates of deinstitutionalization and dehospitalization. Integrated local-based care service packages are designed, including common users db for all services accessible by the operators and the users; and shared caring plans, with user and caregiver access and empowerment, with a single access point for all Cooss services for the user. These packages will involve shared and periodic assessment, case management, information sharing with service buyers (public authorities), and continuity of care, as well as immediate service booking through the online service platform. Also "Social Health Family Learning" courses will be given in collaboration with the Polytechnic University of Marche. These ten-lesson courses will be on specific categories (the first is for congestive heart failure [CHF] patients) and will have the participation of general practitioners (GPs), medical specialists, nurses, social workers, and home care assistants. All the above data are accessible through a shared cross-border platform, and users can decide, when travelling in one of the involved countries, whether or not to make data available to the care provider in the host country. The latest technology available on the market has been tested and some of this technology is integrated in the care process.

14.2   New Care Paradigm for Older People and Older People with Frailty

All agree that demographic changes and aging are a common challenge for Europe. As people age, they are more likely to live with comorbidities (two-thirds of those aged 75+), disability, and frailty. The rising number of elderly people will need different support at home, and they will need different forms of healthcare. At the same time, there is a unique opportunity to bring better health to our older adults, to bring innovative products and services to market, and to establish more sustainable health and care systems. Aging people should be empowered to stay independent, autonomous, and socially engaged for longer within their own homes and communities.

The King's Fund report, "Making our health and care systems fit for an ageing population" [1], argues that health and care services have failed to keep up with dramatic demographic changes. The report finds that transforming services for older people will require a fundamental shift towards care that is coordinated around individual needs rather than around single diseases, and care that prioritises disease prevention and provides support for maintaining independence.

The report authors identify nine individual components of care that needs to improve, with goals that include:

(a) Enabling older people to live well with stable long-term conditions, avoiding unnecessary complications and acute crises;

(b) Improving collaboration between the medical system and social care to ensure that patients can leave hospital promptly once their treatment is complete, with good support available in the community; and

(c) Ensuring that, in times of crisis, older people have rapid access to urgent care, including effective alternatives to hospital. Within the report, the following nine key components have been set out:

    (i) Healthy, active ageing and supporting independence;

    (ii) Living well with simple or stable long-term conditions;

    (iii) Living well with complex comorbidities, dementia, and frailty;

    (iv) Rapid support close to home in times of crisis;

    (v) Good acute hospital care when needed;

    (vi) Good discharge planning and post-discharge support;

    (vii) Good rehabilitation and re-ablement after acute illness or injury;

    (viii) High-quality nursing and residential care for those who need it; and

    (ix) Choice, control, and support towards the end of life.

However, to make all this happen, the key component is that working across teams must be integrated, to ensure that the right mix of services is available in the right place at the right time. There are multiple interdependencies and transitions between components and, in some cases, one team or organization might provide several components.

14.3   Are Changes in Aged Care Leading to Changes in Technology Use in This Field?

According to a survey [2] of 1,200 consumers conducted by Survey Sampling International on behalf of HealthMine, 41 % of consumers have never heard of telemedicine. This number goes up to 46 % for the 45-to 64-year-old group. Overall, 45 % of respondents said they would use telemedicine if it was offered, 16 % said they wouldn't, and 39 % weren't sure. The number who said they would use telemedicine rose to 58 % for millennials (25- to 34-year-olds) and dropped to 37 % for 55- to 64-year-olds. There are no data specific to aged-care technology, but numbers, for sure, are not better. According to Oxford Economics, the so-called longevity/silver economy, which serves the needs of Americans over 50, is currently a $7.1 trillion market and accounts for 46 % of the United States economy (CNBC [3]). As baby boomers age, this niche is forecasted to grow to more than $13.5 trillion by 2032. Baby boomers will be the new disrupters who adopt the technologies, because they expect to live better.

The use of technologies is most likely to be effective in the context of integrated locality-based services designed to support older people, rather than the technologies being used in isolation. The use of telecare solutions should be considered for older people at risk of hospitalization or those moving to long-term care as part of wider integrated-care strategies, and it cannot be assumed that these telecare solutions can be effective without access to a range of other services.

Fig. 14.1 Lively safety watch and in-home hub and activity sensors

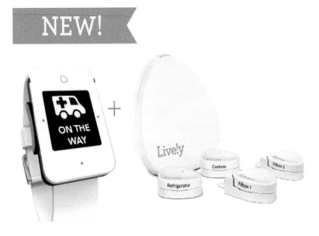

In "Is ambient assisted living the panacea for ageing population?" [4], the main concerns about ambient assisted living (AAL) technology are listed. First is the ease of use for senior citizens (for users with chronic disease, any additional complexity in their lives will increase resistance to using new technologies). Second is the reliability of the proposed solutions (concern about technology malfunctions). Third is aversion to technology and a perceived need for passive systems, with concerns about the effort and cost of installation and maintenance; also, care and technology may be regarded as contradictory terms (often the humanitarian aspect of providing care is believed to be in direct contradiction to the use of technology) (Fig. 14.1).

The design, marketing, and sale channels of aged care devices are changing, and old-fashioned devices are being replaced by new and modern ones. There is no point in a company trying to understand and to respond to the psychological issues of aging if the foundations of its product and supply channels are not fit for purpose for this age group [5].

14.4 The Role of Social Care Providers in Aged Care Technology Development. Cooss Marche User Case and AdriHealthMob Project

There is no best way of integrated care [6]. The lack of integration in planning and strategy causes inefficiencies in service provision. Medium to large operators are trying to fill the gap, making the integration of more services coming from different procurement sources central to integrating the operating side.

Some of the services provided by Cooss Marche are listed in Table 14.1, including the names of service buyers. Although some services affect the same user, there is no data integration and continuity on the planning side. In this situation, Cooss Marche is piloting the integration of local ICT tools, integrating all user data and services in the same platform. Actually the platform is being piloted to be accessed

Table 14.1   Existing situation in local care market and data exchange

Service	Service buyer	Service provider	Real-time data sharing
Home Care	Municipality/Private	Cooss Marche	No
Integrated Home Care	Regional Health Authority	Cooss Marche	No
Protected Homes	Private/Municipality	Cooss Marche	No
Nursing Homes	Private/Regional Health Authority	Cooss Marche	No
Rehabilitation Centers	Private/Regional Health Authority	Cooss Marche	No
Seniors' Tourism	Private/Insurance Funds	Cooss Marche	No

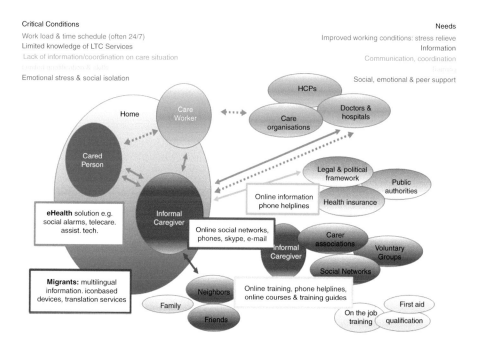

Fig. 14.2   Care Process Map

by operators, users, and their families, but it will be easily integrated on the planning side when this option is made available.

The different actors involved during the home care process are shown in Fig. 14.2 [7]. Based on the situation described in Table 14.1, and considering that telecare services have demonstrated efficiency for patients with cardiac failure, diabetes, and chronic obstructive pulmonary disease (COPD) [8], it appears that

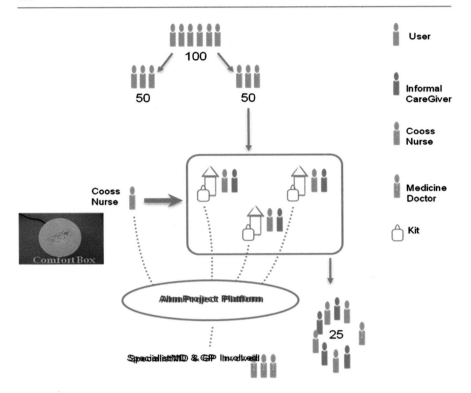

Fig. 14.3 The Pilot Protocol Process

telehealth can play an important role in the delivery of care to remote and rural populations [9]. Cooss Marche has contributed to the preparation and submission of the AdriHealthMob project, in which the Cooss Marche contribution within the project is to demonstrate the piloting of innovative solutions to improve mobility within the care sector, both at the local and cross-border levels.

The pilot protocol is being performed in the Fano area, Marche region, and involves 100 users affected by CHF. An integrated care protocol was agreed upon and is shared by specialist physicians, social care providers, the users, and their families.

A Cooss Marche case manager and a community-based team is coordinated by the local district, where a nurse from Cooss Marche, a specialist physician, a GP, and a social worker participate. Support and education for the family and informal caregivers will be provided during the Social Health Family Learning courses designed and implemented by the Polytechnic University of Marche; to support and empower users to take more control over their health and wellbeing, the next step will be providing the users with access to the AdriHealthMob Platform; all information will be shared under appropriate information governance and respecting privacy rules (Fig. 14.3).

The new protocol and technology will make possible the effective use of the workforce. The key points of the pilot protocol are:

(i)   Specific integrated protocol (user-targeted and including the existing care and medical services provided);
(ii) Provision of home-based passive monitoring kits;
(iii) Provision of operator-assisted medical monitoring kits;
(iv) Provision of environmental monitoring kits (comfort box);
(v)   Social Health Family Learning courses;
(vi) Cross-border mobility of users is considered; and
(vii) User access and empowerment.

The home-based monitoring kits (50), which will be used for everyday self-monitoring, consist of a weighing scale, sphygmomanometer, oximeter, everyday measurements protocol, and journal.

The operator-assisted medical control kits (10) will be used by homecare nurses/nursing home operators; these kits consist of a 12-lead electrocardiogram (ECG) device, tablet computer, wireless sphygmomanometer, and wireless oximeter. Weekly home medical measurements will be submitted by the Cooss Marche nurse.

14.5   Innovative Senior-Oriented Market Technology

Paula Span (in the *New York Times*) creates a picture of innovation in aged care technology. For sure senior-oriented technology is fast becoming more central for the technology world. According to Stephen Johnston, a co-founder of Aging2.0, which connects technology companies with the senior care industry, 1,500 silvertech start-ups had arisen globally in the past 3 years. Which scenario represents the likelier future for senior-oriented technology? It depends on whom you ask. Actually most devices or apps are at the pilot phase and not on the market. The new-generation products and services are considering some basic issues, such as those mentioned below.

The priorities of older adults mirror those expressed by adults of all ages; technology cannot stop the evolution of chronic conditions, but it can improve the quality of life of older people living with their conditions and it can improve their lifestyle. WHO estimates that more than half of the burden of disease in people over 60 is potentially avoidable through changes to lifestyle; assistance in monitoring or adequate treatment for minor needs that limit independence; being included in and being part of care continuity and care coordination; and the involvement of older people and their families in planning and coordinating their own care.

Very useful in orienting users toward aged care technology use is The Family Caregiver's Guide to Electronic Organizers, Monitors, Sensors, and Apps, prepared by the United Hospital Fund [10].

The following is a list of some silver-oriented technology, devices, platforms, and apps already on the market.

   (i) Online basic check up (*Roobrik, BadaCheckUp*);
  (ii) New generation helpline (*Lively*);
 (iii) Remote monitoring (*Lively, Evermind, Onkol, Carepredict, Winmedical, Quietcare, Beclose, Safeinhome, Sense4care, Telemedware*);
 (iv) Online market place, for caregivers/families (*Uber, Honor, Carelinx, Familydea*);
  (v) Integrated (home care + residential care) care services (*Grandcare, Caremerge, Vynca, Vitaever*);
 (vi) Integrated services, medical and care services (*Vitaly-Portal, Santigo-HIS*);
(vii) Tour operator and dating specialized for the elderly (*Adventurra; Stitch*); and
(viii) Hardware PC solutions for the elderly (*Breezie*).

Conclusions

Some aspects we can consider about aged care technology are:

Most of the solutions proposed are stand-alone tech/ICT tools (except for Honor and Uber). There are only a few solutions that are ready to market, mostly coming from the United States market and not fully available in the European Union. United States products are nearer to the market; the user's needs are central, and service providers are involved in the product and market development. Companies that are already familiar with users and manage a huge amount of data are participating in the definition of the market.

Most of the European Union solutions are AAL program pilots, and only a few of them have reached the market. The main promoters are research centers and universities, and service providers are often involved only in the testing phases.

There is a lack of integrated packages, such as those with the combinations of technology + care operators + medical services + laboratories. Solutions tailored for private-based markets are quite complicated to implement in a public-based system (UE (European Union); changing of the buyer from residential care to homecare must be accompanied by a budget shift, data sharing with the involved public actors, and changes in pricing and rules). All solutions so far are part of a too-fragmented market—no Apple and no Google has arisen to integrate this market.

References

1. Oliver D, Foot C, Humphries R (2014) Making our health and care systems fit for an ageing population. The King's Fund, London
2. http://mobihealthnews.com/45492/survey-41-percent-of-consumers-have-never-heard-of-telemedicine/

3. http://www.cnbc.com/2015/10/12/top-vcs-target-7-trillion-senior-care-market
4. D'Angelantonio M, Oates J (2013) Is ambient assisted living the panacea for ageing population? IOS Press, Amsterdam/Washingston DC
5. Straud D, Walker K (2013) Marketing to the ageing consumer. The secrets to building an age friendly business. Palgrave Macmillan, Houndmills/Basingstoke/Hampshire
6. Ham C, Walsh N (2013) Making integrated care happen at scale and pace: lessons from experience. The King's Fund, London, UK
7. Stewart J, Centeno C (2011) JHC Institute for Prospective Technologies Studies. Joint Research Centre - European Commission, Scientific and Policy Reports, 2013
8. Davies A, Newman S (2011) Evaluating telecare and telehealth interventions. The King's Fund, London, UK
9. Goodwin N, Sonola L, Thiel V, Kodner D (2013) Co-ordinated care for people with complex chronic conditions: key lessons and markers for success. The King's Fund, London
10. United Hospital Fund. A family caregiver's guide to electronic organizes, monitors, sensors and apps

ecardioNet: The Role of Electronic Medical Records and ICT in Transnational Projects

15

Antonio Baccan

15.1 Introduction

The ecardionet Project is part of the Programme for European Territorial Cooperation (Italy Slovenia 2007–2013) and aims to build a multiregional cardiology network.

The Local Health Authority 14 (Unità Locale Socio Sanitaria [ULSS] 14) of Chioggia is the smallest health authority in the Veneto Region of Italy, although the city of Chioggia has the seventh highest number of inhabitants of cities in the Veneto Region.

The ULSS 14 is an organic part of the Veneto Regional Health Service, and its mission is to meet the needs and expectations of citizens' health by implementing efficient management of available resources and ensuring the performance of disease prevention and effective care, in a timely fashion, with respect of the person and in conditions of safety.

The Department of Information Systems directed by the writer provides support to the management and all users, of the hospital and territorial, for the appropriate use of information and communications technologies.

The areas of management skills, entrusted to the Operating Unit (UOS), can be divided into three main areas: information systems and networks, application procedures, and analysis and control.

Information systems and networks: This area comprises the corporate network and ServerFarm help desk for computer- and telephone-related areas for internal staff and mmg/pls territory (family doctor territory); landline/mobile data systems; the management of enterprise communications, hardware, and infrastructure; video surveillance security systems; the analysis and design of new infrastructure and

A. Baccan
CIO Local Health Authority 14, Chioggia, Venezia, Italy
e-mail: antonio.baccan@gmail.com

© Springer International Publishing Switzerland 2017
G. Rinaldi (ed.), *New Perspectives in Medical Records*, TELe-Health,
DOI 10.1007/978-3-319-28661-7_15

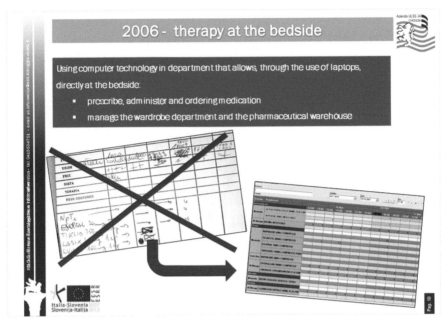

Fig. 15.1 No more paper for the right dose, patient, time and route

technology solutions; European projects; processes of institutional accreditation; and Unit for multi-dimensional evaluation (UVMD) support.

Application procedures: This area comprises the health information system (Medtrak-TrakCare), departmental information systems, and the territorial interfacing of business applications with information technology (IT) adjustment of information systems (IS); the area also includes the regulations and requirements of the strategic direction of the organization.

Analysis and control: This area comprises a data warehouse, and support for company information flows, ministerial and regional information flows, and social and health structures.

UlSS 14 is Veneto's smallest health authority and, because of this, it has focused increasingly on technology to compensate its financial and personnel limits: as an example of its efficiency, the cabling infrastructure of the hospital as well as the corporate email and web browsing systems were activated in 2001.

The ULSS 14 was the first Italian public company (in December 1997) to acquire enterprise resource planning (ERP) software in the health area— Medtrak—which recently underwent technological upgrading, with transition to the web-based version TrakCare. This took place on March 10, 2015, but the flagship application was made in 2006 with the activation of computerized therapy at the bedside.

That procedure enabled clinicians to access the ERP system directly at the bedside, execute orders, and manage their departments in a paperless fashion (Fig. 15.1).

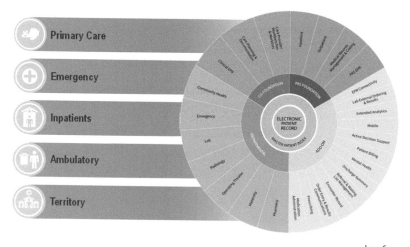

Fig. 15.2 The Electronic Patient Record is the Center of the Information System which ensures an integrated care for the patient

The TrakCare system supports the continuity of care through the integration of five independent workflows: primary care, emergency, inpatient access, ambulatory procedures, and healthcare provided in the territory (Fig. 15.2).

In 2001–2002 a warehouse system for the Chioggia hospital's data was created with the statistical analysis system (SAS), and this was completed in 2014 with the SAS Visual Analytics (VA), which allows accessibility and availability of data and reports; it is truly amazing, and it can also be used on an iPad (Fig. 15.3).

There are, of course, a number of departmental systems specialists who are involved in the corporate network; first of all is Operating unit (UO) Cardiology, directed by Dr. Roberto Valle, who started the whole European eCardionet, as represented in Fig. 15.4.

15.2 The Core of the Cross-Border Project

The project "Model for the prevention of clinical cardiovascular risk in populations of Veneto (Italy) and Obalno-Kraska (Slovenia) from 2004 to 2005", was the first step in the cross-border collaboration. The project, introduced in the European Union (EU) initiative Interreg Italia-Slovenia 2000–2006, concerned the creation of the Point of observation and monitoring of the cross-border map of cardiovascular risk, anticipating synergies between cardiologists and general physicians belonging to the two nations.

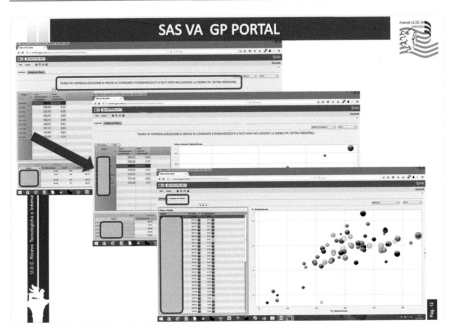

Fig. 15.3 Data warehouse SAS and information portal SAS VA for the management and for family doctors

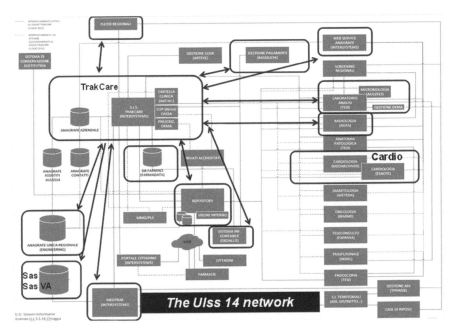

Fig. 15.4 Representation of the company network with the central and departmental information systems

e-Cardionet, following the first experience, was designed by three cardiology departments, those of the hospitals listed below, in Chioggia, Mirano, and Trieste, each of which has a specific role.

15.2.1 Madonna della Navicella Hospital of Chioggia

This department has the role of lead partner. It has developed a program for the implementation of good clinical practice in patients suffering from heart failure, in two phases, namely:

- screening of the local population with coordinated actions by general practitioners (GPs) and health districts, in order to identify all patients in the territory; and
- strategies of intervention to implement all behavioral, dietetic, and therapeutic measures that can positively influence the patient's prognosis, and that can detect early clinical indicators to change the intensity of the follow-up protocols.

An important part of the project was the realization of a system for the sharing of clinical cases "at a distance".

A cardiology picture archiving and communication system (PACS) was also created to store instrumental images and enable collaboration with other Italian and Slovenian partners.

Furthermore, a web portal was set up for the exchange of diagnostic and scientific contributions, in order to build an online library, both for training courses and for health workers involved in the trial.

The decisive factor was the contribution of the partner European Economic Interest Grouping (EEIG) Net Europe Trieste, an entity included in EU law and made up of a cross-border public-private partnership between Italy and Slovenia, which enabled the achievement of results and operability in the territory, through the computerization of the systems, data exchange, and information activities.

15.2.2 Cardiology Department of the University Hospital of Trieste

Because of its strategic location in the area of the program, this cardiology department has developed a plan to improve emergency rescue procedures and the suitable treatment of patients in the border area between Italy and Slovenia.

A technological system of mobile units was created; these units send a patient's data, vital signs, and an electrocardiography recording to the cardiology center, so that, in the hospital, it is possible to set up suitable acceptance measures and the appropriate intervention ready for the patient.

The next steps will be coherent with the program of rehabilitation and disposal established by the host structure with the territorial structure in which the citizen resides.

15.2.3 Cardiology Department of the Local Health Authority 13 of Mirano

This department has proposed an innovative path of rehabilitation that provides a physical exercise program within a multidisciplinary approach.

Patients with chronic heart failure, patients with cardiovascular disease, and those undergoing revascularization with angioplasty are selected.

The program involves a team of specialists and gymnasiums in the area, in which qualified personnel are present, for the administration of exercises, cardiopulmonary resuscitation, and the use of the defibrillator.

The Cardiology Departments of the above Hospitals of Chioggia, Mirano, and Trieste have developed this project with other partners to network the best practices in cardiology, with proper communication and cooperation systems, in order to improve the quality of life of the people in the program area.

Operational protocols were defined, based on the definition and diffusion of quality and quantity standards, with the appropriate use of the technologies and with the creation of an information portal for operators and, ultimately, for the citizens.

15.3   The Electronic Patient Record (EPR) and the Technological System

The core of the project is the implementation of an unified, fully integrated information system based on the EPR of the patient.

Many of today's health information system products are not unified solutions that share a common data repository, so they require the purchase and the implementation of additional products to address interoperability issues – often at high cost and with disappointing results.

The ICT Department has implemented a unified system with seamless modules that use a single high-performance database to store and share all patient records. For this reason, access to the EPR requires just one login for users, and when data is entered it is immediately available throughout the system.

In addition, our unified system facilitates interoperability, with legacy and future applications, because it was built on our advanced integration engine.

The EPR provides analytics tools that are easy to access because they are embedded in its modules. Analytics tools are used for patient records, and for this reason clinicians and managers are able to make fully informed decisions based on complete and up-to-date information.

Real-time management information is provided through reports, graphs, and dashboards. Users see predefined data models and key performance indicators (KPIs) for clinical and administrative data.

The most important feature is the patient-centric design. We believe that well-designed electronic health record systems can improve patient safety while also enhancing productivity. Clinicians provide different information about the patient and each information set is shared with the other clinicians participating in the care.

This approach to complex data management enables clinicians to capture, share, understand, and act on all of their data, leading to better clinical outcomes. So the EPR is oriented around the patient; the patient information is accessible from a single screen. Clinicians use the workflow capabilities to readily view their most important priorities, see outstanding tasks, and collaborate with care teams – improving productivity and reducing the cognitive load.

The database is used for the collection of data on cardiovascular risk factors and their changes upon the application of clinical pathways, with the creation of a web platform that has restricted access for consultations and the insertion of complex clinical cases that can be discussed through videoconferencing connections for teleconsultation.

eCardionet has been able to use the infrastructure built into the e-health strategic plan that has defined the guidelines for access to online services and archives by health workers and the public.

15.4   The Objectives of the eCardionet Project

These are the three objectives in the clinical area:

- Management of heart failure: definition of screening guidelines by cardiologists, family doctors, pharmacists, and controllers, and setting up a cross-border register of heart failure patients; patients are identified with the "drug track" system.
- Process of multidisciplinary care and rehabilitation: guidelines and staff training within gymnasiums; patient enrollment; and monitoring of vital data at the gymnasium.
- Cardiac emergency network in the border area: integration of database (db) telemedicine emergency department with the db (and partners); manual architecture of the new emergency cardiology system; acquisition, installation, and testing telemedicine equipment on mobile vehicles.

The following are the technological objectives:

- PACS treatment of cardiology heart failure, with specific db anonymized equipment for screening (Chioggia);
- Definition of a rehabilitation protocol with a multidisciplinary rehabilitation system for the control and remote monitoring of patients in the gymnasium (Mirano);
- Cardiac emergency network in the border area, with the aim of telemedicine system integration in mobile vehicles and drafting a manual for the use of the system (Trieste);
- Design and creation of a web portal for cardiac area (Chioggia, Mirano, and EEIG).

15.5   The Importance of Cooperative Programs

During the past few years there have been different projects of cooperation between Italy and Slovenia.

These projects have demonstrated the importance of designing integrated information systems that support the clinicians.

At the moment, the technology is dedicated to the implementation of EPRs and the integration of the different medical records systems.

15.5.1 Strategic Project "e-Health" in the Macro-border, as a Project Partner

The e-Health project aims to increase the quality of life through the coordinated development of health and social systems, and specifically the quality of life of Italian and Slovenian patients through new information and communication technology (ICT) tools.

A higher-level system of computer networks connected in a common program was created, in order to equip health professionals with more effective operational tools. This system will allow the development of synergies and interoperability between the health systems of Friuli Venezia Giulia, Veneto, Emilia Romagna, and Slovenia. The system will also develop networking of the healthcare programs of the entire area with the use of ICT tools, with the first trial of the digital and bilingual clinical organization, with telemedicine activities, teleconsultancy, and professional training, as well as language training, in addition to information and communication.

15.5.2 Project Glioma: Project Standard GLIOMA

The project concerns the identification of new markers of cancer stem cells for diagnostic and therapeutic aim, is co-founded as part of the European Cross-Border Cooperation Programme of Slovenia-Italy 2007-2013.

The increased incidence of cancer can be attributed mainly to environmental pollution and incorrect lifestyles. In particular, with regard to brain tumors, an increase has been shown in the incidence of glioblastomas, the histological type of more malignant glioma. These tumors are extremely aggressive and, despite the treatment approaches currently used, the life expectancy of patients with glioblastoma is about 12 months. Glioblastomas are exceptionally resistant to conventional therapies and most modern therapeutic approaches. For this reason, clinicians and researchers must focus their research on the study of new molecular targets and biomarkers, to improve the diagnosis, prediction of responses to treatment and, thereby, also the prognosis.

In particular, this project is focused on the study of the role of cancer stem cells in glioma. Recent scientific discoveries have in fact shown that these cells are responsible for tumor growth and expansion, and probably also for relapses. The results of the activities of this project will contribute to the creation of important new diagnostic instruments, related to canceled improvements in prognosis and prediction of response to therapy, and potentially to new therapeutic strategies.

A joint Italian-Slovenian biobank of tumor samples has already been created and scientific and technological networks will be created, which will enable us to develop international collaborations with institutions and research centers of excellence.

15.5.3 Network Surgical Macro Cross-Border Area, as a Project Partner

The "e-surgerynet" project proposes the creation of a network of excellence for the surgery in border area to apply appropriate models and clinical interventional organization and management.

Cooperation in the multiregional area is useful for sharing new surgical and anesthetic techniques to facilitate the circulation of standard protocols. A common technology platform allows the use of a specialist referral network through live and on-demand sessions, and the creation of and access to a surgical video library—an area of e-learning dedicated to professional training. The creation of a joint network between hospitals promotes the harmonization of social and health services in the program, optimizes the use of existing resources, optimizes professional qualifications, and actions between public and private institutions in applied research, as well as facilitating citizens' access to assistance with measures that improve the overall quality of life. These activities are located in the provinces of Venice and Trieste in Italy and the statistical regions of Obalno Kraška, Gorenjska, and Osrednjeslovenska in Slovenia.

The General Surgery Health Authority 13 of Dolo (Veneto), as lead partner, has made available to other partners their experience in testing new interventional techniques which combine minimally invasive surgery, and intravenous anesthesia performed without gas anesthesia. For the surgeon, clinical protocols in the field of laparoscopic surgery and natural orifice surgery (Natural Orifice Transluminal Endoscopic Surgery) are applied. The anesthesiologist adopts the total intravenous anesthesia-target controlled infusion (TIVA-TCI) technique, where there is only the use of intravenous anesthetic drugs provided by computerized pumps. In this way this procedure offers the surgeon a high quality of work and offers the patient optimal anesthetic induction, maintenance, and awakening.

The Department of Surgery of the General Hospital of University of Trieste has made available to other partners reproducible organizational surgical management models, standardized and exportable for every hospital reality. The protocols so created, approved by the Joint Commission International, are also the result of cross-border cooperation with the Surgical Clinic of Ljubljana and the Hospital of Izola. The principles are to achieve high levels of quality of care, to reduce human error, and to provide logistical support in cases of complications. These principles are particularly related to operative time standards and techniques, card check-in and check-out for the operating room, the use of technological support, and the management of 'fast-track' surgery, from preparation to postoperative course. Other Italian and Slovenian partners will cooperate in the planned activities.

To support research and collaboration between the partners a technological platform was adopted to allow for specialist advice, and to create and provide access to a surgery video library. The system records interventional sessions, allows for the classification and storage of significant contributions, enables the partners to participate in multivideo teleconsultation conferences, and provides open sessions, on request, for further specialized topics. The archived material will form the database that will be used to start distance learning courses for staff. Also on the web portal, partners can enter their contributions, and they can consult the library online by accessing the reserved place dedicated to e-learning.

15.5.4 Project United4Health (U4H)

The project United4Health, UNIversal solutions in TELemedicine Deployment for European HEALTH care, was promoted by NHS 24 Scotland, as coordinator of the same, during the sixth call of the CIP ICT PSP-2012 of the European Commission.

U4H is a European project that aims to consolidate and strengthen the evaluation and deployment of large-scale ICT services for the home treatment of patients with chronic diseases. Specifically studied are people suffering from major chronic conditions: diabetes, chronic obstructive pulmonary disease (COPD), and cardiovascular diseases. The 3-year project started in January 2013 and is based on the experience of European regions of europe working together for health (RENEWING HEALTH), which is characterized by similar goals. The entities subject to validation in RENEWING HEALTH, partners of U4H, have selected a limited number of services that will be tested in 15 European regions to get a sample of data that allows the comparability of results. The Veneto region is represented by ULSS 14 Chioggia, with the technical support of Arsenàl.IT. This consortium is in charge of the design, sharing, and monitoring web platform that collects data from all the pilot areas. The aims of U4H are: to demonstrate that solutions for the treatment of patients with chronic diseases, based on the personal health systems (PHS) under study by RENEWING HEALTH, are transferable to other regions and can be developed on a large scale; to demonstrate that the data collected in RENEWING HEALTH U4H can be the scientific basis for the benefits that such services can provide for people with chronic conditions and their families, as well as providing useful support for professionals who use the services; and to provide economic analysis that highlights the savings that such services generate for the health system.

15.5.5 Love Your Heart Project

The European Love Your Heart project, together with the Adriatic Cardiovascular Diseases Prevention Network, has as its lead partner the Istria Region (Croatia), as part of the IPA Adriatic Cross Border Cooperation Programme 2007–2013.

As part of the IPA Adriatic Cross Border Cooperation Programme, the Love Your Heart project aims to promote healthy lifestyles and start pathways for the qualification of social and healthcare workers. .

Actors: the Istria Region (Croatia), the Central Training School (Italy), ADRA (an Albanian non-government organization [NGO]), and hospitals and healthcare facilities of Istria (Croatia) and Veneto (Chioggia and Porto Viro), as well as consorzio europeo formazione addestramento lavoratori (CEFAL) (which will coordinate the Italian partnership, as an associate member of scuola centrale di formazione (Scf)) will provide actions targeted at education and schools.

Project goal: to improve the health of people, the precondition for any progress, through the creation of a network of cross-border healthcare providers. Specifically, the Love Your Heart project aims to improve the lifestyles of the people through education to create conscious consumption. This aim, with particular reference to food, will involve the training of young people who will work in the catering sector. And, at the same time, this project aims to qualify professionals and facilities in the health system and welfare system through training and sharing best practices, as well as providing certification systems and models of the coordination and integration of services.

Telemedicine in Collaborative Diagnosis and Care of Congenital Heart Malformations

16

A. Taddei, A. Gori, E. Rocca, T. Carducci, G. Piccini,
G. Augiero, A. Ciregia, M. Cossu, R. Conte, G. Ricci,
G. Rocchi, N. Assanta, P. Festa, B. Murzi, and L. Ciucci

16.1 Introduction

Congenital heart malformations represent the foremost birth defect in developed countries (incidence of 0,8 per 1,000 cases per year). Echocardiography is applied for diagnosis and management of these malformations while community hospitals often lack access to pediatric cardiology consultants or sonographers and frequently infants or newborns are transported to a specialized pediatric center. Given the wide-bandwidth networks, interconnecting main health institutions today, it is conceivable to set up low-cost telemedicine services, from tertiary to secondary healthcare centers, providing collaborative diagnosis, care or intervention planning, and follow-up of heart malformations, early in the fetus, in the newborn, or in the child and up to the adult patient.

A. Taddei (✉) • A. Gori • E. Rocca • T. Carducci • G. Piccini • G. Augiero • A. Ciregia
M. Cossu
Heart Hospital/Medical Informatics, Gabriele Monasterio Tuscany Foundation, Massa, Italy
e-mail: taddei@ftgm.it

R. Conte
CNR Institute of Clinical Physiology, Pisa, Italy

G. Ricci
Association "Un Cuore un Mondo", Massa, Italy

G. Rocchi
Lions Clubs International, Pontremoli, Italy

N. Assanta • P. Festa • B. Murzi
Heart Hospital/Pediatric Cardiology, Gabriele Monasterio Tuscany Foundation, Massa, Italy

L. Ciucci
General Manager, Gabriele Monasterio Tuscany Foundation, General Manager, Pisa, Italy

© Springer International Publishing Switzerland 2017
G. Rinaldi (ed.), *New Perspectives in Medical Records*, TELe-Health,
DOI 10.1007/978-3-319-28661-7_16

The "Gabriele Monasterio" Tuscany Foundation (FTGM) (http://www.ftgm. it) (a public healthcare research institution, jointly set up by the National Research Council and Tuscany Region and specialized in cardiovascular diseases) developed a number of projects aimed at health cooperation by telemedicine technology in diagnosis and care of heart malformations involving the pediatric division (Cardiology and Cardiac Surgery) and medical informatics at the Heart Hospital in Massa. Since 2008 the FTGM Heart Hospital, supported by the association "Un Cuore un Mondo" and the Tuscany Region, experienced tele-echocardiography with selected pediatric and gynecology centers in the Balkan countries, from Croatia to Bosnia-Herzegovina, Albania, and Romania [6–8].

Since 2013, jointly with CNR Institute of Clinical Physiology (CNR-IFC), FTGM has been involved in the European IPA Program with the project *AdriHealthMob* (http://adrihealthmob.eu), aimed at developing a cross border model of sustainable and efficient transport services for the health and care sector, in order to improve the mobility of passengers (residents/tourists/users/patients) and to improve accessibility to health and care services [7].

The main objectives include the creation of an area within the Adriatic region of cross border health and care made of connected and interrelated best practices and excellences; the promotion of the ICTs and the enhancement of their potential in terms of eHealth and eCare, as opportunity to reduce (and even "delete") geographical distances, allowing a complete "accessibility"; and the promotion of protocols and memorandum of understanding within the Adriatic area, leading to concrete case of Adriatic cross border health and Adriatic Health and Care Insurance Card.

Fifteen partners of eight countries (Albania, Bosnia-Herzegovina, Croatia, Greece, Italy, Montenegro, Serbia, and Slovenia) were involved. *AdriHealthMob* platform for eHealth and eCare was designed for providing service through distance support for the rationalization of mobility flows up to the elimination of useless transfers for health and care. It deals with telecommunication and distance control among health and care institutions; videoconference facilities for face-to-face contact between users and experts; second opinion and clinical support; and telemedicine to connect hinterland/rural areas with doctors, nurses, and specialists, avoiding mobility and travels.

Among the pilot actions of *AdriHealthMob* project, the empowerment and extension of telemedicine services in collaborative diagnosis and care of cardiac malformations, previously experimented by the FTGM Heart Hospital in Balkan countries, is under development.

Recently (since 2015) a telemedicine network was planned in our region (*"Arriviamo al cuore di tutti" – Telemedicine network for early diagnosis and care of congenital heart disease*) interconnecting neonatology, gynecology, and pediatric centers with the FTGM Heart Hospital, with the financial support of Tuscany clubs of Lions International Association (http://lions108la.it) and of Lions Clubs International Foundation (http://www.lcif.org) as well as with the promotion of healthcare regional authorities.

16.2   Methods

Pediatric tele-echocardiography has been used over many years in various countries, since the first live transmission of neonatal echocardiograms in 1996. Recently, Sable et al. (Children's National Heart Institute, USA) evaluated the impact of telemedicine on delivery of pediatric cardiac care in community hospitals. Telemedicine has the potential to increase efficiency and quality of care, improve echo quality, prevent unnecessary transport of babies without critical heart disease, enhance sonographer skill level, yield financial savings, decrease length of hospitalization, and raise patient and physician satisfaction. There has been a steady increase in the numbers of institutions performing tele-echocardiography [4, 5].

While echography equipment allows recognizing cardiac abnormalities, in neonate or even in fetus, often sonographers are not skilled and live guidance during patient examination is demanded to reach an expert-enlightened joint diagnosis. Thus the synchronous approach is preferred for tele-echocardiography.

Real-time tele-echocardiography was implemented, as in other experiences, by use of videoconferencing technology for streaming echocardiograms over network connections and allowing the specialist at tertiary pediatric center (HUB) to guide the remote ultrasound operator. Basically two CODECs are inter-networked (H323 IP, upload >512 Kbps), the first one in the echography room at remote center and the other one at the HUB (FTGM Heart Hospital in Massa), receiving live echocardiograms for second-opinion evaluation (Fig. 16.1). The video signal is online acquired from echocardiography equipment and transmitted to the specialist workstation. Dual video capability is useful for allowing specialist to interact, during echo examination, with the operator or to interview patient's relatives. Protection measures are applied to information transactions by CODEC data encryption or by use of encrypted network connections (VPN).

Medical-grade connections of telemedicine workstation in the echography room are assured. Even if lossy compression is applied for streaming (e.g., H264), high diagnostic accuracy is usually achieved in clinical practice, as reported in a number of experiences [4, 5, 9].

That approach was applied since 2008 for implementing a cross border network with Balkan countries for real-time pediatric/fetal tele-echocardiography (as described in the following paragraph), while further developments in the other projects provided additional facilities aimed at patient data exchange, image recording, second-opinion reporting, and service management. In order to overcome possible drawbacks in synchronous transmission of echo images, mainly due to lossy efficient compression (H264) and performance instability of public network connectivity, store-and-forward facility (recording high-resolution images on echo-equipment in DICOM standard and transmitting them to the specialist center) was introduced. Revision of evaluations of cardiac malformations by DICOM images, preserving diagnostic information according to telemedicine regulations, was thus allowed achieving definitive second-opinion reporting [3, 7].

An information system (eHealth portal), securely accessible over public network, allows to share patient clinical data for thorough second-opinion evaluation

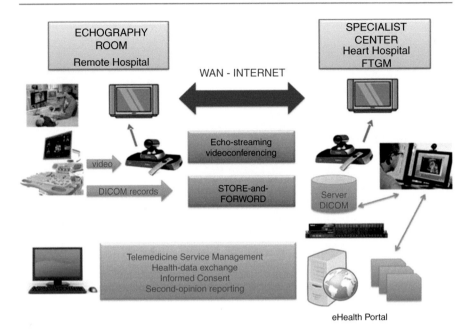

Fig. 16.1 Tele-echocardiography system for collaborative diagnosis of cardiac malformations: videoconferencing is applied during examination for guiding the operator and later DICOM images are transferred for revision and second-opinion reporting. The eHealth portal provides facilities for secure data exchange and documentation of telemedicine service

as well as reporting. Formatted reports with digital signature will be provided. Generally, the physician, who examines the patient, is charged of writing the echocardiography report taking into consideration the second-opinion evaluation of the specialist. Actually according to the protocol of the Tuscan project, the report should be unique, just signed by the two physicians, cooperating by telemedicine.

Finally, tele-echocardiography is a two-step process (as represented in Fig. 16.1):

- Firstly, synchronous tele-echocardiography is achieved by streaming echo low-resolution (compressed) images during videoconference, so allowing remote guide for proper exploration of cardiac anatomy.
- Secondly, at the end of the examination, high-resolution DICOM images are transferred to the specialist center, directly from the echography equipment or from the hospital imaging system (PACS), for allowing revision/confirmation of diagnostic evaluations and second-opinion reporting.

Within the AdriHealthMob project, a central eHealth and eCare web portal will be provided, while in the Tuscan Lions/LCIF project (Arriviamo al Cuore di Tutti), the FTGM information system facilities have been made available by proper adaptation for creating a medical outpatient record for both data sharing and diagnostic reporting.

Particular attention was dedicated to learning for allowing fruitful at-distance collaboration in pediatric or fetal echocardiography. Initial learning of medical staff is planned by stages at the Heart Hospital while videoconferencing facilities are conveniently used during the project. Technical guides for telemedicine use and troubleshooting were initially provided by FTGM technicians, which have been continued cooperating to assistance at remote centers throughout the activity.

In AdriHealthMob, CNR-IFC was charged of providing the remote learning platform (RLP) for professionals. In accordance with the other partners of the project, CNR-IFC, in collaboration with the FTGM Heart Hospital, will provide a basic echocardiography course on congenital heart disease. RLP is composed of two main components:

- The e-learning application: containing all data needed to acquire knowledge in a specific domain (based on open-source Moodle software for remote learning) (www.moodle.org)
- The e-training application: implementing the programs to improve own knowledge and skill in a specific pathology, by means of evaluations on real clinical studies (web-based tool developed by CNR-IFC in order to improve participants' skills in image interpretation)

16.3   The Balkan Network

Since 2008 the Pediatric Cardiology and Cardiac Surgery teams of the Heart Hospital of FTGM in Massa, supported by Medical Informatics researchers and jointly with the volunteers of "Un Cuore un Mondo" Association, were involved in the International Health-Care Cooperation program of Tuscany Region. The goal was to set up a cooperative network with the clinical centers in Balkan Countries for supporting the diagnosis and care of congenital heart malformations [6, 8].

Tele-echocardiography was first implemented at Pediatric Clinical Centres of Banja Luka (BIH) and Rijeka (KR), at the Gynaecology Hospital in Tirana (AL). Later other centers in Bosnia-Herzegovina (Gynecology Hospital/Sarajevo and Pediatric Hospitals/Tuzla and Mostar) as well as in Romania (Bucharest) were involved. A telemedicine network connecting the remote clinical sites in the Balkan Area with the cardiac department of the Heart Hospital in Massa/Italy (the reference center) was set up over the Internet (Fig. 16.2).

Videoconferencing equipment (Aethra Vega ×3/×5) was applied, for implementing real-time tele-echocardiography. Standard audio/video interaction was provided between the clinicians in Massa and the sonographers/physicians at the remote Balkan sites. Echocardiograms were performed under the remote guide of pediatric cardiologists from Massa. The video analogue output of the echocardiography equipment was connected with the CODEC (Fig. 16.1) for image acquisition/digitization and efficient data compression allowing transmission in real time by standard H.323 protocol on IP network. Upload data transfer rate, greater than 512 Kbps, was provided to ensure quality and low latency of transmitted echocardiographic images.

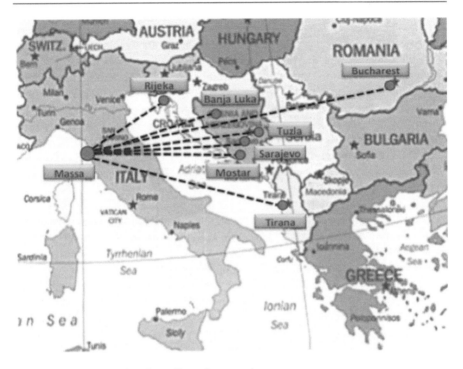

Fig. 16.2 The Balkan tele-echocardiography network

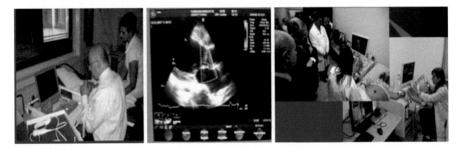

Fig. 16.3 Pediatric (from Banja Luka) and fetal (from Tirana and Sarajevo) tele-echocardiography (*left* to *right*)

At the Heart Hospital in Massa, the echocardiographic images were decompressed and displayed for teleconsulting.

Real-time tele-echocardiography was implemented at both pediatric and gynecology (Fig. 16.3) centers. Real-time teleconsultation helped to plan timely care or intervention in case of critical or complex conditions, even transferring pregnant women before delivery in case of fetal abnormalities. Standard cryptography was applied for data protection. At times, limitations of public network bandwidth (the Internet), or instability of it, affected quality of diagnostic images and the degradation was high enough to render detection of cardiac abnormalities difficult. In these situations store-and-forward solution was applied as alternative, transferring imaging records (possibly in DICOM format) thus preserving diagnostic information.

Patients with suspected heart malformations were evaluated on-demand by tele-echocardiography from pediatric cardiologists at the HUB in Massa assessing the abnormal or critical cases. In the last years, 82 patients (29 neonates, 30 infants, and 23 children) were transferred from Albania, Bosnia-Herzegovina, and Croatia for cardiac surgery. Each patient or fetus was first examined by tele-echocardiography in most of the cases. While a part of them were evaluated not complex, minor, or normal, the others were transported to Massa for cardiac surgery intervention or care. Even pregnant women, in case of critical fetal abnormalities, were transferred before delivery to the birth center in Massa to allow prompt intervention on newborns for limiting risks. Follow-up of patients, going back to home, was facilitated by the use of the network.

Videoconference meetings and workshops were organized for discussion of clinical cases and for training healthcare personnel. Nevertheless, adequate exploitation of the network requires refining the cooperation agreements with the hospitals, which were not really active, thus promoting wide cooperation in health care in the Balkan area.

16.4   AdriHealthMob

The EC IPA *AdriHealthMob* (*AHM*) project (Adriatic model of sustainable mobility in health and care sector) (http://adrihealthmob.eu) foresees the participation of 15 partners from the 8 countries that constitute the macro-Adriatic region. By the involvement of institutions, universities and research organizations, public and private stakeholders in the health sector, and ICT companies, a partnership was established aimed at developing guidelines, through research and pilot actions, for a sustainable transport strategy to ensure the citizens an easy access to health services. FTGM Heart Hospital jointly with CNR-IFC is contributing to activity work packages, particularly involved in the extension and empowerment of previous telemedicine experiences in cardiac malformations.

FTGM and CNR-IFC research teams are involved in developing a pilot service in collaborative diagnosis and care of heart malformations through the *AHM* ICT network.

As described in the methods, the remote learning platform, designed by CNR-IFC, will be experimented, uploading significant cases of heart malformations, cared in FTGM Heart Hospital [1].

Next, after initial training on site, the enrolled centers (up to nine from the different participating countries) in the Adriatic area will be provided with RLP for acquiring or extending knowledge for ultrasound examination of cardiac malformations.

The tele-echocardiography network will consist of the enrolled centers, all networked across the *AHM* portal platform with the hub centers (FTGM/Massa and others). Each center is equipped with a workstation acquiring echo images from echography equipment (Fig. 16.1) and streaming them to a specialist center for second-opinion evaluation. The eHealth and eCare *AHM* web portal, implemented by the ICT partner company, will provide services for requesting consultations, patient data sharing, and second-opinion reporting. DICOM images will be stored into a server for documentation and revision. Recently, technical solutions for providing both second-opinion evaluation and real-time echo streaming have been designed and proposed to the AHM project partnership.

The pilot action will start after workstations for tele-echocardiography have been installed and tested. The results of 1-year experimentation will be analyzed and reported.

16.5   "Arriviamo al Cuore di Tutti": LIONS/LCIF Telemedicine Network for Early Diagnosis and Care of Congenital Heart Disease

In Tuscany (region in central Italy with three million inhabitants, comprising a couple of major islands), some thousands of patients each year (including pregnant women) are traveling for diagnosis and care of cardiac malformations to specialized centers (FTGM Heart Hospital in Massa and Meyer Hospital in Florence). This project (Fig. 16.4), developed by FTGM with the financial support of Lions Clubs of District 108La Tuscany (http://lions108la.it/) and of the Lions Clubs International Foundation (http://www.lcif.org/) and with the promotion of Health-Care System of Tuscany Region, is implementing tele-echocardiography network interconnecting at least one at each of its ten provinces, with priority for remote locations, not easy for traveling (Fig. 16.5).

Pilot action started at the Hospital of Elba Island: tele-echocardiography was tested successfully connecting the cardiology lab with the pediatric department of Heart Hospital in Massa through a secure network (VPN) (Fig. 16.6).

Echocardiograms, under the guide of the specialist, are streamed for detection and evaluation of cardiac malformations. A portable telemedicine cart has been assembled to facilitate use within the hospital. First, the telemedicine service has been started at Elba hospital (Fig. 16.6). Later, at the hospitals in Lucca, Empoli, Pontremoli, Bibbiena and Arezzo (Fig. 16.7), telemedicine workstations have been installed, while others will be set up within the next year throughout the region (beginning from Prato, Pistoia and Versilia). The Meyer Hospital in Firenze will be involved as second HUB of the network. According to current development plans up to 15 pediatric/neonatology sites will be connected in order to cover the full region. Official agreements have

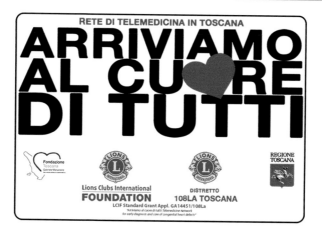

Fig. 16.4

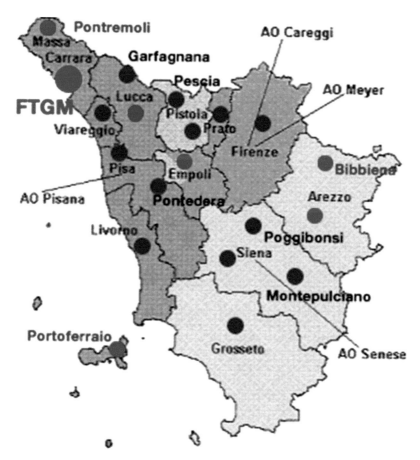

Fig. 16.5 The telemedicine network, developed by LIONS/LCIF "Arriviamo al Cuore di Tutti" project, will interconnect all main pediatric/neonatology centers around Tuscany with the HUB consulting center (FTGM and later Meyer Hospital)

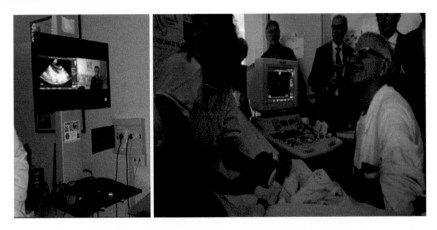

Fig. 16.6 The telemedicine cart applied for teleconsultation from Heart Hospital in Massa during echocardiography examination on neonate at the Hospital of Elba Island in Tuscany

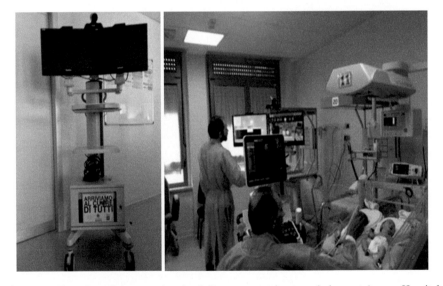

Fig. 16.7 The telemedicine cart (on the *left*) was set up in neonathology at Arezzo Hospital including the following: videoconference equipment is connected with digital video output of echocardiography instrumentation (on the *right*); two monitors are provided: one for videoconferencing and the other for medical reporting. All inputs are medically insulated

been signed by FTGM with Health-Care Institutions to deliver telemedicine services. According to the functional layout of Fig. 16.1, the "live" tele-echocardiography session is followed by the transmission of DICOM records to FTGM server for revision, while a medical record system (running on FTGM server) is securely provided for

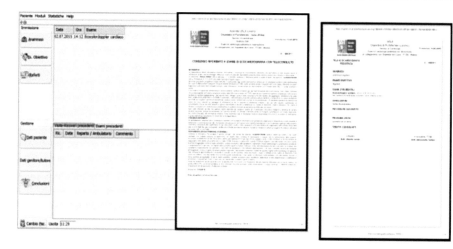

Fig. 16.8 Medical record system for documentation of examinations is provided (by remote VPN access to FTGM clinical information server). From *left* to *right*: the graphical user interface including commands for patient data entry (anamnesis, physical examination, test reports, relatives or tutors, conclusions) and printing visit report with diagnostic evaluation as well as informed consent according to legal constraints

documenting clinical conditions and for preparing a report, agreed by both the physician, caring for the patient, and the specialist colleague. Information document and informed consent are also provided to respect legal constraints (Fig. 16.8).

Conclusion

Tele-echocardiography allows collaborative medical decision making in diagnosis and care of complex and critical heart defects. It plays an important role in the early diagnosis, follow-up, or exclusion of cardiovascular abnormalities, planning patient mobility to tertiary specialist center when really necessary. Quality and continuity of care are provided with overall cost reduction avoiding unnecessary patient transfers, examinations, or hospitalizations. Continuous medical training at secondary centers is also achieved.

The main benefits of telemedicine network are:

- Shortening the time to diagnosis limiting risks for patient
- Preventing unnecessary patient transports and avoiding discomforts for families
- Promoting a real pediatric network, empowering the medical skill out of specialized centers
- Extending specialized remote consultation for follow-up of patients undergoing high-specialty interventions
- Reducing costs for both families and the public health systems

Videoconferencing technology, by wide-bandwidth networking, is promoting diffusion of low-cost telemedicine networks in the study of various medical pathologies, just providing specialized medical care virtually anywhere.

The added value of the cross border cooperation in the *AdriHealthMob* project relies in the implementation of interoperable network for health and care services. Cross border cooperation will allow to improve transport routes for health and care as well as to promote the development and networking of health and care resource in the Adriatic area. The most recent developments on eHealth and the newest mHealth (MobileHealth), together with the directive on cross border health in Europe, confirm how innovations in health and care can influence the transport and mobility schemes as well as the quality of services provided. In the framework of health and care (as well as for transports), services fall within the scope of several legal instruments and legislative framework, asking for agreement, protocols, and procedure; with a view to implement an integrated transport, health and care system, the cross border cooperation will contribute to:

- Clarify areas of legal uncertainty.
- Improve interoperability between systems.
- Increase awareness and skills of target groups.
- Promote initiatives of health (digital and road) routes.
- Ensure legal advice for start-up eHealth business

Expected results are:

- Improvement of accessibility and mobility in health and care sector by simultaneous operational actions on innovation and ICT introduction on one side and on Adriatic regional planning on the other
- Full knowledge of mobility and transport schemes for health and care; introduction of systems for permanent and systematic collection and analysis of data and statistics
- ICT-driven models for the optimization and rationalization of cross border mobility for health and care
- Driving implementation of electronic patient summary, ICT Resource Centre, and platform for eHealth and eCare
- Networking capacity to implement services of telemedicine (tele-assistance/diagnosis/consultation) leading to Adriatic cross border health care
- Strategy for sustainable transport for health and care, based on joint, integrated planning in the Adriatic area

Permanent tool for policy and decision makers, the Adriatic Health and Care Mobility Association (AHCMA), to plan health and care, to network providers, and to identify integrated funding schemes

Acknowledgments We thank for their collaborative efforts the clinical and technical teams of centers participating in the Balkan project, particularly Prof. V. Ahe (University of Rijeka – School Medicine), Dr. R. Moisiu ("Koco Gliozheni" Gynecology Univ.Hospital – Tirana), and Dr. S. Bajic and Dr. D. Djukic (Pediatric Clinical Centre, Banja Luka). Thanks to "Un Cuore un Mondo" Association and their president Mr. M. Locatelli for financial support jointly with Tuscany Region. Moreover, we thank Dr. Ilir Qose for continuing collaboration in the management of the AdriHealthMob IPA project. Finally, as concerns the project for telemedicine network in Tuscany ("Arriviamo al Cuore di Tutti"), thanks to Lions Clubs of the District 108La (Tuscany) and to the Lions Clubs International Foundation (LCIF) for financially supporting this project; special thanks to Dr. Gianluca Rocchi, District 108La Governor (until June 2015) of Lions Clubs Association, for promoting and supporting the development and implementation. Also, thanks to the clinical and technical teams of Health-Care Institutions around Tuscany for the great support to develop the telemedicine network (particularly dr. Iurato, Azzarelli, Zipoli, Cozzalupi, Marri and Martini). Thanks also to Dr. Alberto Genova for the legal advice in the definition of informed consent and protocol agreements and Dr. Maurizio Mangione for his advice in development of medical record system for reporting telemedicine examination.

References

1. Bansal M, Singh S et al (2015) Value of interactive scanning for improving the outcome of new-learners in transcontinental tele-echocardiography (VISION-in-Tele-Echo) Study. J Am Soc Echocardiogr 28(1):76–87
2. http://adrihealthmob.eu (the portal of the AdriHealthMob project). Accessed 20 Oct 2015
3. Italian Ministry of Health. National Telemedicine Guidelines. http://www.salute.gov.it/imgs/C_17_pubblicazioni_2129_allegato.pdf. Accessed 20 Oct 2015
4. Krishnan A, Fuska M, Dixon R, Sable CA (2014) The evolution of pediatric tele-echocardiography: 15-year experience of over 10,000 transmissions. Telemed e-Health 20:681–686
5. McCrossan BA, Grant B, Morgan GJ (2008) Diagnosis of congenital heart disease in neonates by videoconferencing: an eight-year experience. J Telemed Telecare 14:137–140
6. Taddei A, Carducci T, Gori A, Rocca E, Assanta N, Festa P, Djukic D, Bajic S, Murzi B (2008) Tele-echocardiography between Italy and Balkan area. J Cardiovasc Med 9:S20
7. Taddei A, Gori A, Rocca E, Carducci T, Piccini G, Augiero G, Ciregia A, Murzi B, Festa P, De Lucia V, Ait_Ali L, Assanta N, Ricci G, Rocchi G, Ciucci L (2014) Telemedicine network for collaborative diagnosis and care of heart malformations. Eur J Prev Cardiol 21:S2
8. Taddei A, Gori A, Rocca E, Carducci T, Piccini G, Augiero G, Festa P, Assanta N, Ricci G, Murzi B (2014b) Telemedicine network for early diagnosis and care of heart malformations. In: Lacković I et al (eds) The international conference on health informatics, IFMBE Proceedings 42 – Springer International Publishing, Switzerland, pp 268–271
9. Triunfo R, Tumbarello R, Sulis A, Zanetti G, Lianas L, Meloni V, Frexia F (2010) COTS technologies for telemedicine applications. Int J CARS 5:11–18

Health Dossier in Italy: Elements for Reflection, What's New, What Are Possible Improvements

17

Fabrizio L. Ricci and Angelo Rossi Mori

17.1 Introduction

In recent years, the European Union and therefore also Italy are calling for a new healthcare attitude in response to the strong growth of health needs and increase of related issues; the demand goes beyond healthcare and invests on the quality of life. Healthcare must be seen by a systemic approach: sharing and continuity of care, new organizational models enhanced by information technology and telemedicine, and so on.

The new modalities to deliver social and health services for primary care should be read in this context: (a) a citizen-centric approach based on clinical pathways, (b) the improvement of collaboration among healthcare facilities, (c) integration of health and social care, and (d) quality improvement of physician activities.

The response of the Italian healthcare system is slow and inefficient, highlighting not only a misuse of resources but also high costs of the system due mainly to waste. A more appropriate use of information and communication technology (ICT) would allow a better response in terms of a more efficient use of resources and of delivery of services and therefore to increase productivity in the assistance and in the prevention, as well as a reclassification of expenditure: the advanced information management can be an opportunity to improve the healthcare system, putting the citizen at the center, to ensure their quality of life, to respond flexibly to diverse needs of people, by personalized home care [1].

LAVSE (Virtual Laboratory for eHealth) is composed of various researchers from different institutes of the National Research Council (CNR), Italy.

F.L. Ricci (✉) • A. Rossi Mori
LAVSE, CNR, Rome, Italy
e-mail: fabrizio.ricci@cnr.it; arossimori@gmail.com

© Springer International Publishing Switzerland 2017
G. Rinaldi (ed.), *New Perspectives in Medical Records*, TELe-Health,
DOI 10.1007/978-3-319-28661-7_17

Therefore, a new model of information management is required, for example:

- Health providers need more and better information in order to simplify access to and share of health information on a specific patient, guidelines, epidemiology, and so on.
- Patients need to simplify access to information about (a) their own health status, (b) guidelines and better lifestyles, and (c) services guaranteed by law.
- Health managers need more and better information for more efficient resource use and effective clinical service delivery.

The long-term trend is the implementation of a common information substrate for all the actors and for all types of needs, as is already happening successfully in some organizations more cohesive and efficient (i.e., Kaiser Permanente, Maccabi) [8]. This implies a shared vision among the various actors working in the healthcare system; it means that we need a method for the first stages of analysis of a complex project of eHealth, able to generate a framework in which the eHealth solution is harmonious and sustainable (suitable for clinicians and patients), respectful of citizen privacy.

The method was used to analyze the FSE being implemented in the Italian regions. FSE (in Italian "Fascicolo Sanitario Elettronico" = Electronic Health Document Folder) is a new electronic service implemented for all citizens in a jurisdictional area as a region, for storing the clinical documents generated during clinical contacts carried out in a facility or by a health provider during a visit with a citizen [15]. A Working Group composed of researchers of LAVSE-CNR and the Italian Association of Telemedicine (SIT) has used this method to propose how the FSE may go beyond the current limits. The aim of this Working Group was to define the requirements of an evolution of the FSE in order to innovate the processes of healthcare, research, education, and governance for raising the quality of services and improving the health and social well-being of citizens.

17.2   A Method for Analyzing the Innovative Healthcare Models

Social and healthcare must be viewed with a systemic approach as a response to new challenges [7]:

- Continuity of care, especially for people with long-term needs, such as the chronically ill and vulnerable people; in particular for Chronic Care Model, disease management/integrated management, active and healthy aging, the enrollment of patients in aging various forms of home care programs
- Models of collaborative working among professionals (groups of GPs, multiprofessional groups) and new types of the facilities (e.g., primary care centers)
- New professional profiles, such as care managers (i.e., nurse navigator in the USA), a nurse with the role of helping citizens and caregivers to manage the care plan agreed
- Making citizens more responsible about their health (patient empowerment, patient engagement, adherence to the care plan agreed)

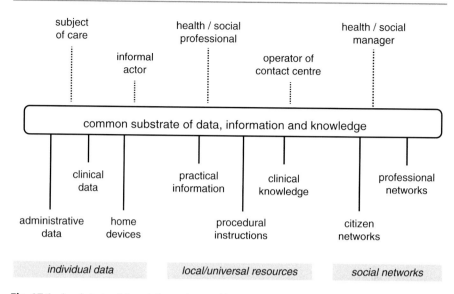

Fig. 17.1 A substrate of data, information, and knowledge, shared by all actors, which are agents in the health system

- Secondary uses of routine data, appropriately coded for the calculation of indicators and the construction of dashboards for the government system and the self-assessment of the health providers

The ICT may be a tool that facilitates these changes; in order to provide the appropriate information, it is necessary to point out the most important aspects of integration as a basis for planning information management [12]:

- Integration of decision-making tasks (administrative, organizational, and operational) and the related documentation
- Integration among different settings of care delivery, particularly between hospital and primary care
- Integration among the actors, including not only formal carers but also the citizen and his caregiver, in a "functional team" made from time to time (implicitly or explicitly) in function of the patient's needs
- Integration among the health problems of the individual patient, in a holistic view, also as integration between health and social care
- Integration between the ICT solutions and medical devices (both for the measurement of clinical parameters that support for the non-self-sufficiency, such as home automation), to carry out structured activities
- Integration of structured documentation and informal information/communication

As indicated in [11], this implies the construction of a substrate of data, information, and knowledge, shared to all actors, which are agents in the health system (see Fig. 17.1). For specific situations interleaving, a platform is created. In Italy the FSE can play a role, whether it will be able to respond to the real needs dictated by the use of clinical information and their reorganization.

To arrive at a design for a platform, we need to have a holistic view of the tasks to which they are called upon to perform the application software needed to support the professional activity of the potential users of platform/application software.

In the case of the FSE, this means that the FSE should be a support system in the creation and management of a collaborative environment (configurable from case to case) for the definition, planning, enactment, and retrieval of a social and health workflow of a patient and to allow secondary uses of these data and in particular the evaluation of the results of care pathways.

Therefore, to define a platform, we need to have a holistic view of the majority (at least the most important) business process that the application software running on it must support. This means that the business scenarios of the use of the platform are needed to be defined. So for the definition of the requirements of the platform, the following activities must be carried out:

- *Analysis of use cases* – it is a common technique used to find out the functional requirements of a software system; a use case provides the objective that a user wants to achieve with the system.
- *Case histories* – through the narration of some scenes (which accurately describe the events from multiple points of view), we have the bottom-up definition of the use cases.
- *Interviews* – we want to survey the perspectives of the opinion leaders; these perspectives could be considered as top-level use cases.
- *Analysis of literature* – it means access to the public knowledge of the use case.
- *Analysis of rules and laws* – in healthcare, there are various legislative constraints that delimit the course of the use case.
- *Analysis of experiences, foreign and specifically Italian* – this is the theme of good practices but also the analysis of potential failures.

For example, to define the requirements of the FSE, we systematically analyzed the main use cases (considering as reference the national guidelines by the Italian Ministry of Health, which suggests the areas of application of the FSE):

- *Continuity of care based on shared care pathways* – this use case relates to the provision of care services and continuity of care between different structures and health providers, also including aspects related to prevention and risk factors, as in the case of treatment of chronic patients.
- *The social and health integration* – this use case involves the connection with social services, i.e., all services that provide better quality of care addressing them in a holistic view.
- *The involvement of citizens in the management of their own health* – this use case implies proactive citizen and therefore all services to facilitate its accountability in the management of health.

- *Operational and administrative services* – this case is related to all those services (e.g., prescriptions, medical reports online, certificates) that are carried out in relation to assistance and who are not strictly clinical.
- *Use secondary information* – this case focuses (but not exclusively) on governance, epidemiology, and scientific researches.

17.3   The Main Requirements for a Platform for the Integration of Social and Health Care

The "health" of the citizen, according to the WHO, should be considered in a holistic perspective of quality of life: (a) managing the complexities of the disease, (b) integration of health and social services provided by different structures, (c) active collaboration of the citizen, and (d) equitable access to health services [5]. In the continuity of social or health assistance, the functional team (which explicitly or implicitly works with a citizen on his plan of care) must behave as a coherent system in front of the citizen, despite physical dispersion in the territory. The caregiver and the citizen may be considered as members of the functional team for the management of the activities planned in the treatment and assigned to the improvement of lifestyles.

17.3.1 The Continuity of Care

The continuity of care is based on the coordination among the various activities and therefore requires (a) the selection and stratification of patients to identify the care pathway to be applied; (b) the adaptation to the context of the reference path, to get the care plan of the individual patient; (c) the education of the patient about his condition; (d) active monitoring of the health status of the patient in order to intervene promptly if necessary; (e) the consistent management of the shared care plan; and (f) the management of home medical devices.

It is necessary to regulate and to support mechanisms to raise the mutual awareness of the functional team around the citizen, by means of an explicit formulation of the caregiving agreement, accepted by the citizen. It is suitable to share knowledge about the mandates of care of each health worker or health facility (whether it concerns a total or partial takeover, whether it is temporary or permanent), with the role, objectives, and duration.

It is necessary to enable systems for processing the data generated by the equipment home managed by patients and caregivers; in this manner health provider can operate when specific predefined events happen. The platform should provide the basic software, whose orchestration can implement value-added services, making up the Electronic Assistant Professional, for example, early warning systems, tools for online discussion of the single clinical case, and so on.

17.3.2 The Social and Healthcare Integration

The social and healthcare integration allows to address the issue of quality of care in a holistic manner. It should also consider (a) the influence of the social context of the patient and his caregiver on the execution of the plans of care and (b) the promotion of the autonomy of the citizen and the integration of people at risk of marginalization. This means that social providers should (a) help improve adherence of citizens to the individual care plan, (b) support the citizen in his daily activities (clinical, social, relational, etc.), and (c) support the citizen to manage the administrative and operational tasks [6]. In fact in the care of a chronic patient, the most critical services are (a) education for managing their own health, (b) the stimulus to a better adherence to the treatment plan, and (c) removal of the time lost in administrative steps. We will then think about the design of an electronic assistant to the caregiver.

17.3.3 The Patient Empowerment

The patient empowerment means a citizen involvement in the management of their own health, and it is therefore necessary to facilitate its activation: the personal health system goes in this direction [2]. Therefore, one should (a) strengthen the self-care management, (b) facilitate collaboration among citizens and health providers, and (c) ensure the monitoring of health status and the progress of therapies. For this reason, we need to help the citizen to move along three guidelines: (1) functional (understand health information), (2) critical (process information acquired), and (3) integrated (share information and interact with patient groups and associations). The aids are numerous and some are already present, even if not in a vision enabling their integration: they are available as commercial products, for example, alarms, diaries, medication dosage calculation, telemonitoring systems, and so on [6].

It should be noted that it is not enough to plan a series of actions in some way educational, informational, motivational, and others to foster a proactive citizens but must be studied a complex strategy that takes into account all the factors and all the players involved; otherwise, there is the possible failure of the entire operation [3]. In fact the risk of abandonment is "substantial" as well as that of nonacceptance by the medical staff.

17.3.4 Operational and Administrative Services

The objectives are (a) to facilitate and streamline operations for the citizen (which is especially felt in rural or mountainous areas) and (b) to plan more effectively the delivery of health services or synchronize, in real time, the various activities carried out by the various actors in a functional team. In fact, during the execution of a care pathway, different interlaced processes (operational, administrative, and managerial) are activated; we should plan to activate, execute, and monitor the various phases of the management processes that underlie the execution. Various bureaucratic procedures (e.g., certificates) are present.

However, information on the state of the administrative management procedures (such as change of bookings, details of the procedures performed, temporary unavailability of a patient's home) are information of rapid obsolescence: they must be managed for a time restricted (e.g., they are deleted after a time interval defined) to be lighter on the system.

17.3.5 Secondary Uses of the Information

The FSE could be an opportunity to implement a systematic collection of data (appropriately coded) related to interventions carried out; we have a basis (a) to build pathways to care based on evidence, (b) to study the risk factors, (c) to allow for programming of resources and the optimal allocation of the same, and (d) to process data for research purposes [10]. Information objects should be structured in a standard way, according to a cumulative data dictionary (on clinical, health, and social data). The absence of codes on many variables makes it difficult to aggregate data from heterogeneous information systems. This is achievable today only in limited areas (e.g., on a single disease and a specific care pathway): a general approach is needed. For frequent situations, relatively stable and predictable, you can have timely indicators calculated from routine data.

For secondary uses of the FSE, we have to define metadata and associations between concepts in the right way to allow better use of the data and a better search; it should be noted that the information objects are to be represented in such a way to be processed according to precise semantic standards (coded name of the variable, the list of allowed values, units, explicit, etc.). This way you can create a data warehouse.

From the point of view of *governance*, management systems for managers can be readily powered by integrated and reliable information, extracted from routine data, and organized along care pathways' reference; in this way, it is possible to assess the appropriateness of the resources compared to the specificities of individual patients.

From the point of view of *epidemiological surveillance*, it is possible to prepare the reporting of sentinel events: the timeliness of reporting and, in the long run, the completeness of the coverage of all health structures of a judicial area (e.g., city) make it a tool potentially essential. The availability of a huge amount of data detailed and structured, from the routine processes of care, allows us to define the progress of disease and to study the effectiveness of assistance.

From the point of view of *scientific research*, availability of data collected routinely during clinical events during the entire life of a citizen (expanded with additional relevant data and links to external databases) can offer (a) the basis for the sizing of clinical trials in the third stage and (b) the identification of new predictive factors (especially if there is a connection with bioimaging and with a connection tomorrow with omics data).

Like all systems of management of clinical information, there is the opportunity to use the FSE to support the *professional training*. A system of management clinical information could be a good source of real patient stories to extract cases for educational purposes. It provides an overview of the healthcare status of an individual to support professionals in the delivery of care services. It can be considered a repository of real clinical cases, also deployable in their temporal complexity, usually without any explicit statement about the logic of the decision process. The extraction of health case studies from it for educational purposes must therefore take into account the needs defined above and allow the learners to practice a) identifying the essential information and the points of decision; (b) taking autonomous diagnostic, therapeutic, and management decisions; (c) comparing their decisions with those actually made in the reality of that particular case; (d) balancing the rationale of their decisions with the available scientific evidence, collected from knowledge bases; and (e) discussing their work with a tutor.

17.4   FSE: Limits and an Evolution Suggested

The Working Group[1] of LAVSE-CNR and SIT on FSE analyzed limits and suggested an evolution. The questions of Working Group were:

- Does the current platform address the needs or will it be a flop?
- Which value-added software services can make FSE more useful?
- How to integrate the information more closely related to the quality of life?
- Which FSE role develops an economy that pays more attention to the citizen's needs?

One element of these questions is also the good deployment of the FSE.

The results of this Working Group were a manifesto (see Appendix) and a book [9]. The aim of this book is to put the thoughts on how the actual FSE was designed and implemented and what should be the characteristics of a more comprehensive architecture, of which the FSE is only one of many elements.

To achieve these results, the Working Group has applied the method of use cases described above; these use cases were analyzed from the following points of view: (a) basic features, (b) administrative and operative view, (c) technological view, (d) bottlenecks of the actual and foreseen FSE, and (e) main problems and possible advices.

---

[1] The members of Working Group on FSE are:

- LAVSE-CNR: Isabella Castiglioni, Daniela Luzi, Gregorio Mercurio, Carmelo Militello, Fabrizio L. Ricci (coordinator), Angelo Rossi Mori Oscar Tamburis, and Rita Verbicaro
- SIT: Maurizio Cipolla, Mario Costa, Antonio V. Gaddi, Velio Macellari, Marco Manca, Michele Martoni, Chiara Rabbito, Giulio Rigon, Giovanni Rinaldi, Giancarmine Russo, Giacomo Vespasiani, and Luigi Zampetti.

The FSE, defined by the Italian Ministry of Health, is "the digital set of medical data and documents generated during clinical present and past events related to a citizen, through all his/her life"; it is a longitudinal (lifelong) electronic record for all citizens in a jurisdictional area as a region [10]. It is a software platform able to manage a collection (not well structured and not exhaustive) of clinical documents (in standard format by CDA/HL7), the use of which mimes the manual paper-based management; the documents (containing a collection of information on the patient's health, collected during a clinical event) can be shared between all regional health information systems.

A big problem of the health system is the lack of integration between the various actors in the system (territory and the hospital). These actors do not share patient data in a continuum of care: the response of the FSE is to make available electronically signed documents (according to a document-driven approach), but its metadata (author, date of issue, document type, point of care) describe it without taking into account the context (e.g., missing the problem that originated the clinical event, in relation to which the document was created).

With this in mind, some critics are related mainly to the following missing aspects: (a) managing data extracted from documents stored in the FSE and their processing, (b) criteria for organizing information such as linking documents (and the data in them) to episodes of care and clinical events, (c) the need for a pervasive use of international standards, and (d) infostructure semantics that allows the structured representation of the concepts and be processed in the FSE (data, clinical pathways, and so on).

Another mistake is to consider the FSE as an "infrastructure," to support the management of individual healthcare professionals, the systems for the management of hospital medical records of the team, and the tools that will assist citizens in self-care. We need to start from a different information latform in which the FSE is a key element of care, prevention, and health education, dedicated to the patient, with data utilizable from the patient himself. The FSE does not duplicate information and even organizational models, but shares the information and makes it available in a format understandable to the patient and allows the introduction of a new contribution of the patient that can complement what is produced by providers.

In order to create a connected health, a federated platform is necessary, where the collaborative work is expressed through providing and sharing of information and through the exchange views in order to reach a common understanding. This information can be used profitably by health providers (including the patient). These providers can also belong to different institutions with different organization models; they also have different goals and different perspectives while working within the workflow of activities shared [11].

In an evolved FSE (nFSE), the basic components of the services for continuity of care (to build the connected health) are:

- Management of assistance mandates (i.e., the composition of the functional team) and profiles of the actors

- Management of notifications of relevant events, filtered according to the role and profile of each actor
- Management of shared and harmonized patient's health issues and problems

The components mentioned above will assume a more intense value if connected to a series of ICT services ICT (present in nFSE) allowing to define the care path suitable not only for the clinical problems but also or the social ones.

An nFSE must behave, along with other support tools, not only as a source of information but also as a valuable aid in the creation and management of a collaborative environment configurable from case to case, for patient centric care systems. The nFSE must be able to support the work of health workers and patient empowerment and to allow the secondary uses of their data and in particular the evaluation of the results of the care pathways. For example:

- To determine the disease or condition that explains the patient's symptoms and signs, a care provider can look for information in the nFSE during the diagnosis process. The present in nFSE can navigate in the medical guidelines related to the health issue and provide suggestions for treatment focusing the attention focused only on the details of the care plan.
- The caregiver can also receive notifications about significant events during the course of patient care.
- A manager in the institutional settings of social and healthcare will generate a dashboard decision by analyzing a subset of data extracted adequately.
- With the help of the nFSE, demographic analysts can complete their study of morbidity regarding the incidence and prevalence of a disease during a certain period and/or in a geographical area.
- A patient can view the trend of his/her vital signs measured by healthcare providers (i.e., blood, urine) in recent months and be reminded of a scheduled check or when to take a prescribed medication and also notified of adverse events after administration of a drug.
- A social worker will work together with the health provider for patient care not only in helping with paperwork but also in offering personal services that will decrease considerably the risk of marginalization of the most vulnerable people.

The early evolution of the FSE concerns the change of structure of information: we go from a structure centered on the documents (citizen → document) to a centered on episodes of care (citizen → episode of care → contact → document), where the episode of health or social care is composed of a time-ordered set of social and health contacts that a citizen has with one or many health and social providers (or structures) in order to solve in his/her health or social problem.[2] Thus, the information needed for each citizen are (a) demographic and administrative information; (b) information for emergency situations; (c) clinical event grouped into episodes, each one marked by a health problem (with related mandate); (d) health status marked by sign and clinical observations (qualitative and quantitative) and by the previous but

---

[2] The concepts to be used are those modeled in the standard ContSys (ISO-CEN EN13940:2007).

still active diagnosis; (e) active care workflow described by pathway both already executed and to be made; and (f) digital documents (not only formal) generated by health providers and marked by the different steps of their life cycle (open, closed, deleted, etc.). There are clinical information objects related to definition, planning, enactment, and retrieval of a care workflow, from different points of view (diagnosis, therapy, rehabilitation, social assistance, and so on).

The nFSE has to be oriented to meet "the needs of the citizen, the patient, health professionals, and governments" like all applications of ICT in harmony with the general principles of the European Union on eHealth [7]. In the holistic view of health (according to WHO definition), the "nFSE is a tool of the citizen that can help improve the quality of life for himself, his family and the community" [9]. FSE is a tool of health and social providers. They use this tool according to technical and scientific knowledge as well as their responsibility, adapted to patient's needs. The nFSE is an ICT platform, above which different value-added software services are implemented, acting on health and social sphere [9].

The value-added service, which is based on the nFSE, must arise from a joint and multidisciplinary development of organizational models and technological solutions that take into account the holistic view of the process in terms of coproduction and sharing of data and the activities of any other interconnected processes. The design of a value-added service should be conducted in an environment like living lab and in an environment of open innovation (not indoor research laboratories), in real-life situations. The living lab is based on a systematic user co-creation approach integrating research and innovation processes. These are integrated through the co-creation, exploration, experimentation, and evaluation of innovative ideas, scenarios, concepts, and related technological artifacts in real-life use cases. Such use cases involve user communities, not only as observed subjects but also as a source of creation. The value-added software services for clinical application must be subjected to evaluation of the clinical risk with results made public: it is very important in the case that these software systems are designed specifically for the citizens.

The widespread adoption of FSE and of related value-added services should be guided by following a well-defined roadmap managed by a cabin with strong political power and decision-making. The adoption process should be developed so that the FSE is used daily in real situations for the solution of some problems connected with other high-impact problems, addressed in a holistic way, based on a virtuous relationship among citizens, doctors, and professionals involved. The adoption must be supported by adequate awareness campaign that has to understand the advantages and possibilities of the FSE to the citizens. Adoption is inextricably linked to programs of training and retraining of personnel at all levels to provide adequate professional preparation and a proper approach to the resources of eHealth and thus also to the FSE.

17.5 Conclusions

A platform for supporting the shift from organization-centric to patient-centric model of healthcare service delivery to facilitate collaborative, multidisciplinary, and cross-organizational healthcare delivery processes (together with the Internet of things, telemedicine, mHealth, and so on [4]) is the basis for realizing a health digital ecosystem that interacts with the healthcare system for better supporting it [13, 14]. The agent-oriented paradigm emerges as a promising approach to map the autonomic healthcare systems and their users in virtual entities and to add values such as flexibility, adaptability, and reusability over traditional object- or service-oriented approaches [13].

17.5.1 It Should, However, Make a Preliminary Observation

Dedicated funding to single interventions even if coordinated *are not enough*. If the policy and culture substrate are not mature, *insuperable difficulties* arise in the implementation. In fact, the modernization of healthcare sector requires significant organizational changes in a systemic vision with the support of ICT.

Conditions necessary, although not sufficient, are (a) availability of an adequate numbers of innovators and (b) consensus of stakeholder communities on a shared vision and a common path.

Acknowledgments This work is inspired by the book [9]; our thanks go to the members of the Working Group of LAVSE-CNR and SIT on FSE.

Appendix: The Manifesto and LAVSE-CNR and SIT on FSE [9]

1. *The FSE is a citizen's tool that helps in improving the quality of his/her life, of his/her family, and of community.*
2. The FSE is a tool of health and social providers. They use this tool according to technical and scientific knowledge as well as their responsibilities, adapted to patient's needs.

The Significant Use of the FSE
3. The FSE promotes the proactive role of the citizen, even through the presence of dedicated services to enable them to (a) monitor the health and development of therapies, (b) improve the lifestyles, (c) strengthen the self-care management, and (d) collaborate with more consciously with health and social providers.
4. The primary value of the FSE is the ability to stimulate an environment that works with citizens and health and social providers, coordinating and interconnecting the different types of processes that act on the patient to give rise to a global process of social and health services. To this end the FSE facilitates the management and sharing of information by all professionals, also assembled in functional groups, in the context of care pathways shared.
5. Secondary uses of FSE for purposes of clinical governance, epidemiology, scientific research, vocational training, health education, and proper allocation of resources are reconciled with the main aim to improve the management of individual and community health and to reduce the burdens of bureaucratic-

administrative, managerial and organizational tasks, as well as control of productivity and spending.

The FSE in the Context of eHealth

6. The FSE supports the other tools of eHealth for health management and is interoperable with them; as all systems connected to the health protection, it is consistent with (a) the Constitution, (b) the definition of health of the World Health Organization, and (c) general principles on the health of the European Union, including cross border aspects of care and freedom of treatment.

7. Each value-added service based on FSE must (a) join the interests of the population, the potential of the industry world, and the skills and achievements of scientific and technological research; (b) be designed and implemented in an environment like living lab through a joint development of multidisciplinary organizational models and technological solutions; (c) take into account the holistic view of the process in which fits in terms of coproduction and data sharing and the activities of any other interconnected processes; and (d) be subjected to evaluation of the clinical risk with results made public.

The Adoption Process

8. The widespread adoption of FSE and related value-added services (a) follows a well-defined roadmap managed from a control booth with a strong political decision-making and (b) develops in such a way that the FSE is used primarily for the solution of problems connected with other high-impact problems, addressed in a holistic manner, based on a virtuous relationship between citizens and concerned professionals.

9. The adoption must be supported by (a) an awareness campaign directed at citizens about the benefits and the opportunity of the FSE and (b) training programs and staff training at all professional levels in order to provide an adequate preparation and a correct approach to resources of eHealth.

The Content

10. The FSE manages the object information necessary to the definition, planning, implementation, and historicizing of a care plan in the context of prevention, diagnosis, care, rehabilitation, and social health. These information objects concern data, complex information, warning, and the discussions of clinical case, structured according to a precise dictionary of cumulative clinical and social and health data.

11. The FSE enables the management of individual data, clinical and nonclinical, so as to allow them to connect semantically between them and other information; the data (a) can be processed according to precise semantic standards, systems of encodings, and terminology subsidiaries; (b) are associated with attribute definitors/associations (metadata) appropriate to allow a better and intelligent use of data and a better research; (c) are shared with the candidate applications to use them, developed according European standards; and (d) are relating to documents that contain them in order to interpret its context.

12. The model of the concepts underlying the processes, the standard of integration of interoperability, and coding systems are developed and adopted at national, European, and international level, in accordance with the output from the respective authorities.

13. The information object present in the FSE and necessary to a medical doctor or a social and health provider to carry out social and healthcare activities and assistance can be stored in the same system of the structure in which the staff works, even if generated elsewhere; the storage of any information object relative to the patient must comply as expressly authorized by the latter and is associated with the storage of the information required to be able to trace, within the FSE, the document that contains the element in question.

14. The information collected for purposes not social or health, even if they are tied to the assistance of the citizen (especially if at risk of rapid obsolescence), can be managed in a different system than the FSE, such system must be interoperable to all levels with the FSE, and the information flows must be interwoven with the related information flows of the FSE.

Privacy
15. The FSE must ensure, in any application, the respect of the protection of personal data, professional secrecy and its declination practices, technical measures of security, and guidelines and indications coming from the Authority for the Protection of Personal Data.

16. The FSE must facilitate its use for purposes of scientific and epidemiological research, reworking the information without causing any damage or limiting the protection of personal data. The flow aimed at boosting the FSE will be fully subject to the discipline on the treatment of personal data and the resulting information requirements and collection of consent; it is necessary to provide methods and timing of anonymization of information which would implement the feed flow of the data warehouse, in accordance with the principles that govern the protection of privacy.

References

1. Bulik RJ (2008) Human factors in primary care telemedicine encounters. J Telemed Telecare
2. Detmer D, Bloomrosen M, Raymond B, Tang P (2008) Integrated personal health records: transformative tools for consumer-centric care. BMC Med Inf Decis Making
3. Enos N, Enos M (2013) Three EHR-related coding errors to avoid. MGMA Connexion/Med Group Manag Assoc
4. Free C et al (2013) The effectiveness of mobile-health technology-based health behaviour change or disease management interventions for health care consumers: a systematic review. PLoS Med
5. Gaddi A, Capello F, Manca M (Eds.) (2013) eHealth, care and quality of life. Springer

6. Gu Y, Day K (2013) Propensity of people with long-term conditions to use personal health records. Stud Health Technol Inf
7. Hamilton C (2013) The WHO-ITU National eHealth strategy toolkit as an effective approach to national strategy development and implementation. Stud Health Technol Inf
8. Nazi KM, Hogan TP, McInnes DK, Woods SS, Graham G (2013) Evaluating patient access to Electronic Health Records: results from a survey of veterans. Med Care
9. Ricci FL, Gaddi, Rossi Mori A, Russo G (Eds.) (2014) Verso il Fascicolo Sanitario Elettronico: elementi di riflessione (Toward Electronic Health Dossier: food for thought). RA edition, (in Italian)
10. Rinaldi G, Gaddi A, Capello F (2013) Medical data, information economy and federative networks. The concepts underlying the comprehensive electronic clinical record framework. Nova Science Publisher
11. Rossi Mori A, Mercurio G, Verbicaro R (2012) Enhanced policies on connected health are essential to achieve accountable social and health systems issue on 'Policy lessons from a decade of eGovernment, eHealth & eInclusion. Eur J ePractice
12. Rossi Mori A, Mazzeo M (2013) Holistic health: predicting our data future, from inter-operability among systems to co-operability among people. Int J Med Inform
13. Serbanati L, Ricci FL, Mercurio G, Vasilateanu A (2011) Steps towards a digital health eco-system. JMI
14. Tamburis O, Rossi Mori R, Mangia M (2011) The LITIS conceptual framework measuring eHealth readiness and adoption dynamics across the healthcare organizations. Health Technol, Spring
15. Tang PC et al (2006) Health records: definitions, benefits, and strategies for overcoming barriers to adoption. J Am Med Inform Assoc

The Role of Telemedicine and EHR in Supporting Care Pathways in the Management of Chronic Illness: The Experiences of the Lombardy Region

18

Loredana Luzzi, Gabriella Borghi, Chiara Penello, and Cristina Masella

18.1 Introduction

The world has changed: now it is connected, digitally, socially, iteratively, immediately and personally. Today's digital age is filled with volatility, uncertainty, complexity and ambiguity (VUCA).[1] The world of healthcare is increasingly finding itself having to deal with this reality and taking advantage of the opportunities offered by e-health to address the challenges that are arising, particularly in managing chronicity and fragility.

As stated in the conference conclusions on the EU Summit on Chronic Disease: "Today, chronic diseases affect more than 80 % of people aged over 65 and represent a major challenge for health and social systems. 70–80 % of healthcare budgets, an estimated € 700 billion per year, are spent on chronic diseases in the European Union".[2] In response to the emergency represented by chronic diseases, it is essential to develop and promote clinical pathways, encourage self-monitoring, promote

---

[1] Passmore, O'Shea, and Horney, "Leadership Agility: A Business Imperative for a VUCA World, People and Strategy, Volume 33, Issue 4-2010″Kail, Leading in a VUCA Environment, HBR Blog Network, November 3, 2010 through January 6, 2011.

[2] http://ec.europa.eu/health/maor_chronic_diseses/docs/ev_20140403_mi_en.pdf.

L. Luzzi (✉)
ASST Grande Ospedale Metropolitano Niguarda, Milan, Italy
e-mail: loredana.luzzi@ospedaleniguarda.it

G. Borghi
Cefriel, Milan, Italy

C. Penello
Region of Lombardy Welfare General Directorate, Milan, Italy

C. Masella
Politecnico di Milano, School of Management, Milan, Italy

© Springer International Publishing Switzerland 2017
G. Rinaldi (ed.), *New Perspectives in Medical Records*, TELe-Health,
DOI 10.1007/978-3-319-28661-7_18

appropriate lifestyles and help patients to understand their symptoms and how they can be treated. It is now broadly agreed that these tools for patient empowerment can reduce or delay the deterioration of the patients' functions, limit the worsening of symptoms and reduce hospitalisations.

In recent years, the Region of Lombardy has explored different organisational and clinical solutions to these issues, mostly based on out-of-hospital care. The most interesting experiences, which we are about to describe, took place under a new regional law approved in August of this year.[3]

The goal of the reform is to address the needs of society, above all the ageing of the population and the increased incidence of chronic diseases, while keeping in mind the need to cut costs. The reform envisages the evolution of a regional health-care system in which the focus of political action is how patients are enrolled, the way to integrate treatments and citizens' freedom of choice, and a system that is going to experiment with new organisational and administrative models. This represents a dramatic change over the existing situation. The national government views the regional act and the experience of Lombardy as an experiment that it will be watching carefully over the next 3 years.

The new regional law incorporates a number of elements demonstrating the region's focus on management of chronic diseases:

- It confirms the decision to use CReG (chronic related groups) as a comprehensive fee for managing patients with chronic diseases (art. 5).
- It assigns the new Health and Welfare Companies (*Aziende Socio Sanitarie Territoriali*, or ASST) the task of accepting conditions of chronic disease and fragility as part of an integrated procedure (art. 7).
- It states that the Healthcare System in Lombardy (*Sistema Sociosanitario Lombardo*, or SSL) will "implement innovative organisational methods for accepting patients that are capable of integrating different means of responding to the needs of people in a condition of chronic disease and fragility, partly through use of the latest technologies and methodological practices, particularly telemedicine, so as to ensure continuity of access to the service network and the appropriateness of the medical, health and social services provided" (art. 9).

What follows is a description of what the Region of Lombardy has done in recent years, from the creation of the health information system (*Sistema Informativo Socio Sanitario*, or SISS) in the late 1990s to the more recent experience of the local hospital units (*Presidi Ospedalieri Territoriali*, or POT).

This paper will look specifically at:

- The existing healthcare information system as a new development of the SISS
- The services offered by the New Healthcare Networks (*Nuove Reti Sanitarie*, or NRS) for the remote monitoring of patients affected by CHF and COPD

---

[3] Regional Act no. 23, August 11, 2015.

- The experience of chronic related groups (CReG), a GP-led integrated service for chronic patients
- Local hospital units (POT), small local hospitals that have been redesigned to provide medium- to low-intensity health and welfare services

18.2   Model for Implementation of Electronic Healthcare in the Region of Lombardy

In the mid-1990s, when healthcare was reformed in Lombardy by Law 31/97, the region's entire information system was reorganised to put the citizen at the centre of the health information system (SISS). In architectural terms, this means organising the collection and subsequent processing of data on the basis of the services used by citizens. The Information System in Lombardy now has a data warehouse (DWH) containing administrative data, which allows patients to be displayed in clusters, while the electronic health record (*Fascicolo Sanitario Elettronico*, or FSE) contains clinical data displaying the individual patient's situation.

The electronic health record (FSE), already used by six million people in Lombardy, is the "set of digital data and documents generated by clinical events present and past for a particular patient".[4] Its goal is to provide a unified overall view of the person's state of health. It contains information on medical events and summary documents, organised in a patient-centric hierarchic structure that permits browsing among clinical documents generated by the healthcare system at different times. This promotes quality and appropriateness of care and the upcoming pharmaceutical file will improve compliance with the prescribed treatment and, therefore, protect the patient's safety. The FSE facilitates the provision of healthcare services, making it possible to:

- Oversee the patient's care, permitting better coordination and continuity of treatment.
- Facilitate acceptance of chronic diseases, because it permits sharing of the clinical information required to ensure continuity of treatment among all the healthcare workers involved in the healthcare process.
- Guarantee compliance with uniform rules (such as respect for privacy)

The minimum content of the FSE is defined at the national level to permit exchange of information on patients, and its application is currently evolving at the regional level. In Lombardy, the FSE includes not only information in PDF format but also structured information (HL7-CDA2), particularly for pathology networks, in order to permit more analytical processing for the purposes of monitoring, assessment and planning at the regional level.

---

[4]Law no. 221 of December 17, 2012, no. 221. Conversion into law, with amendments, of Decree Law no. 179 of October 18, 2012, containing additional urgent measures for the country's economic growth.

The FSE may also include diagnostic, treatment and care programmes (*Percorsi Diagnostico Terapeutici Assistenziali*, or PDTA), which are becoming increasingly important. For the chronically ill patient, they represent a tool for ensuring continuity of care and application of the guidelines. They may be identified as "a predefined, articulated and coordinated sequence of services provided in the clinic, during a hospital stay and/or at the territorial level, with the participation of a number of different specialists and professionals (in addition to the patients themselves), with the aim of obtaining the most appropriate diagnosis and treatment for a specific pathological situation".[5] The FSE in Lombardy also includes an Individual Care Plan (*Piano Assistenziale Individuale*, or PAI) and a care pact for patients participating in the CREG project, as described in detail below.

The information contained in the regional information system offers a valid source of support for management of chronic diseases but it is important to pay attention to the quality of information flows. At present, apart from the most consolidated information, the data is frequently expressed in different forms, even within the same institute.

There are two challenges to be faced in the immediate future:

- Making the regional information system increasingly accessible by simplifying interaction processes and taking advantage of new developments in technology (i.e. conduct transactions, and even give orders, using the mobile network)
- Improving the quality of the data collected in order to permit sharing of chronic disease treatment results between different facilities and regions, drawing on information with comparable content.

18.3   New Healthcare Networks (*Nuove Reti Sanitarie*, or NRS)

The New Healthcare Networks provide a framework in which most of the successful projects dedicated to chronic and post-acute conditions have been collected, centrally managed and evaluated, in order to facilitate the process of making them part of routine practices. As shown in Fig. 18.1, the New Healthcare Networks were established in 2006, inheriting the Criteria and Urban Plan for telemedicine for heart failure, to which the protocols created under the Telemaco project for telemedicine for BPCO and specialised teleconsulting services for MMG were added in 2010.

Specifically, the patient management protocol developed in the research projects was proposed as an experimental service to all healthcare facilities in Lombardy that were interested in it and met the requirements for use of the service. A sort of accreditation process was then applied to those hospitals. An experimental fee was then defined and paid on the basis of records submitted through the regional information system. These records were intended to be similar to those used in clinics,

---

[5] Definition taken from the 2010–2012 National Waiting List Management Plan (*Piano Nazionale per il Governo delle Liste d'Attesa*, or PNGLA).

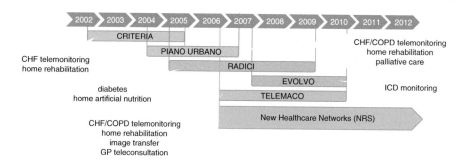

Fig. 18.1 Successful projects merged into the framework of New Healthcare Networks (NRS)

but integrated with the information required to permit monitoring of at-home activities. This is without a doubt the distinguishing feature of NRS experimentation in the years 2006–2011: all processes were assessed every 6 months, and the results of the assessment were presented and discussed with the healthcare teams involved. The analyses regarded aspects such as the clinical characteristics of the participating patients, service indicators, the duration of the processes and causes of dropping out. There was a special focus on customer satisfaction, measured with questionnaires used to detect any criticalities.

When the experiment finished in 2012 and the services went into operation, this form of accompaniment was suspended, but the complete information remained, allowing the region to conduct periodic checks of the work.

The NRS now permits the following services to be provided at home for chronically ill patients: (i) chronic heart failure telemonitoring (PTS) and (ii) home telemonitoring for chronic obstructive pulmonary disease (COPD) patients (PTP).

The services manage at home patients in a serious condition, by integrating the activities of the general practitioner (GP), for a time span of 6 months. The main goals of the services are to reduce the number of hospitalisations and emergency access for heart failure or COPD, to reduce requests for outpatient services, to stabilise the clinical conditions of patients and prevent any instability or exacerbation and to improve the patients' quality of life. The patients receive structured tele phone support with a multidisciplinary care approach referring to medical/nursing interventions made over the telephone. Patients assigned to the PTS or PTP receive (in many cases before hospital discharge) a portable device that uses a fixed or mobile telephone network to transfer data to a receiving station, where a nurse or doctor is on duty 24 h a day, 7 days a week. The technological aspects are supervised by service providers chosen directly by the single hospital, which must meet requirements set by the Region of Lombardy.

The features of these two processes are summed up in Table 18.1.

Data from the use allows us to state that the New Healthcare Networks provide a sufficient at-home response to the healthcare needs of patients with medium to

Table 18.1 Summary of NRS pathways for chronically ill patients

Home telemonitoring service name	Diseases addressed	Technologies	Number of patients enrolled (December 2014)
PTS – Home remote surveillance (since 2006)	Cardiology Heart Failure (II-III-IV NYHA)	ECG single lead set up on the patient	3.731 patients
			35 hospitals
PTP – Home remote surveillance (since 2010)	Pneumology COPD (III–IV GOLD)	Oximeter on the patient	1.987 patients
			31 hospitals

Technologies – Service centre with web-based medical record
Duration – Max 6 months
Experimental tariff – € 720/6 months – € 480/6 months low intensity
Informative flux – Record on regional central informative debt

severe chronic pathologies.[6] Certain pathologies, such as heart failure and COPD, can be dealt with at home even in the most advanced stages with the support of very simple telemedicine systems aided by an organisation that forms a network of physicians, nurses and service providers.

18.4   Chronic Related Groups (CReG)

CReG is a GP-led integrated service for chronic patients. It provides a classification scheme to categorise chronic patients into clinically significant classes, which differentiate the amount of resources required to provide care to patients affected by chronic diseases outside the hospital. CReG was launched as a trial project in the Region of Lombardy in 2012, with the involvement of five health organisations.

The CReG model is based on four pillars[7]:

- A system for classification of patients on the basis of the chronic nature of their illness, identifying patients affected by "chronic" pathologies through algorithms that "read" institutional information flows using "tracers" such as drug use, appointments with specialists, hospital stays and/or fee exemption for certain pathologies.
- A payment system that, like the DRG system, assigns a rate to categories of similar pathologies (or groups of pathologies). The so-called responsibility fee is a predefined amount of resources paid to a single service operator. As in a DRG system, payment is therefore predefined and paid to the operator for accepting the patient in their territory.

---

[6] Giordano, A. et al. – Home-Based Telesurveillance Program in Chronic Heart Failure: Effects on Clinical Status and Implications for 1-Year Prognosis, Telemedicine and E-Health, 2013; 19 (8): 605–612.
   Vitacca, M et al.- Home-based telemanagement in advanced copd: who uses it most? Real-life study in Lombardy - COPD: Journal of Chronic Obstructive Pulmonary Disease, in press.
[7] Region of Lombardy, DGR X/1465 of June 3, 2014.

- The individual care plan, which takes into account co-morbidity and the "real" consumption scenarios described in a list of expected services (*Elenco Prestazioni Attese*, or EPA).
- An all-inclusive method for acceptance of chronically ill patients. The CReG involves active patient management through new operators (GP Cooperatives), which coordinate and supervise the diagnosis and care process described in the individual care plans.

The CReG model is based on an information system that makes it possible to have information available on acceptance of chronically ill patients by GP Cooperatives, which act as "CReG Managers". The regional platform permits digital signature of a "care pact" stipulated between the CReG operator (the cooperative) and the patient, that is, a sort of official agreement that allows the patient:

- To consent to participation in the CReG project
- To become familiar and agree with the content of the individual care plan prepared by his or her GP
- To give specific consent to processing of his or her personal data

By the end of the first CReG trial (2012–2013), 484 MMGs had been involved (7.2 % of all MMGs present in the Region of Lombardy), and 61,901 patients had been enrolled.[8] The results of the preliminary analysis revealed a link between enrolment in the CReG trial and a reduced number of visits to the hospital (emergency ward and ordinary hospital stays), though this must be verified in the follow-up stage[8].

18.5   Local Hospital Units (*Presidi Ospedalieri Territoriali, or POT*)

The local hospital unit was first created in Lombardy in 2013[9] in response to the need to reorganise the hospital network, assigning a number of small hospital sites a role more appropriate to current requirements. In an additional measure,[10] the region identified the local hospital unit as one of the "new forms of organization that will acknowledge the importance of addressing all the needs of chronic patients, planning and organizing personalized healthcare programmes to ensure continuity in diagnosis, treatment and rehabilitation". The regional government set a number of limitations on the opening of local hospital units, such as the requirement that "projects presented must exclusively involve the conversion of *existing accredited*

---

[8] Region of Lombardy DGR X/1465 of June 3, 2014.

[9] DGR X/1185 of 2013: *A bold step towards taking care of the chronically ill, therefore, begins with the establishment of a **separate territorial pole capable of offering its own services and attracting patients as an alternative to the hospital** and which, along with the hospital, will form a virtuous circuit of continuity in the territory.*

[10] DGR X/1521/2014.

facilities, and not the accreditation of new facilities", confirming the fact that the project represented a "reinterpretation" and adaptation of the existing hospital network rather than the creation of yet more service centres.

The interesting thing is that the regional government did not set out to propose a single structural model as a reference but to encourage submission by the health authorities of projects developed for different kinds of individual facilities, in order to take advantage of existing opportunities in the local area that were consistent with the goals of the programme.

By way of example, services that local hospital units can provide include:

• Hospitalisation (beds for subacute patients)
• Day hospital services, including both complex clinical activities and low-intensity surgical macro-activities
• Clinical services, such as clinics of general practitioners, 24-h clinics, specialists' clinics, rehabilitation clinics, nursing clinics, first aid stations, etc.

POT can also provide first-level diagnostic services, such as X-rays, ultrasound, point of care testing, etc., as well as services for the care of chronic diseases (chemotherapy, dialysis, etc.). Local hospital units are therefore destined to "become the functional node of a network of services for the process of diagnosis and care of chronically ill patients, even for the most complex and problematic illnesses requiring repeated check-ups to prevent imbalances. These facilities must be equipped with everything required to provide services necessary for treating chronic patients, other than at times of emergency or acute illness. For example, these facilities must be equipped for taking samples, must be capable of supplying basic specialized services for diagnosis, care or rehabilitation, must directly supply drugs, and/or must guarantee supervision of telecare and telemedicine services".

Regional Act 23/2015 (art. 7) confirms the role of local hospital units as multi-service facilities for providing medium- to low-intensity health and welfare services for patients with acute and chronic diseases. The local hospital unit may represent the physical site of synthesis between patient management by the GP and "direct" management by the local hospital unit, depending on the intensity of care required and the experience of the "New Healthcare Networks". This set-up is summed up in the polygon in Fig. 18.2 representing the chronic nature of disease.[11] This polygon classifies chronically ill patients according to the degree of severity of the chronic illness and underlines the models for acceptance and management of such patients, with the resulting different uses of technology. A recent measure[12] of the regional government defines the method to be applied to determine the rates, the payment agreement and policies for primary care agreements, so as to permit the effective start of work in local hospital units.[13]

---

[11] Regione Lombardia, Libro Bianco – luglio 2014.

[12] DGR X/4191 of October 16, 2015.

[13] The local hospital units approved in 2014 are Sant'Angelo Lodigiano (LO), Somma Lombardo (VA), two polyclinics and Villa Marelli in central Milan, Soresina (CR), Calcinate (BG), Leno and Orzinuovi (BS), Morbegno (SO) and Vaprio d'Adda and Bollate (MI).

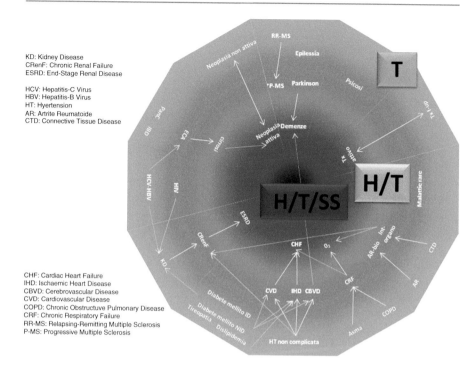

KD: Kidney Disease
CRenF: Chronic Renal Failure
ESRD: End-Stage Renal Disease

HCV: Hepatitis-C Virus
HBV: Hepatitis-B Virus
HT: Hyertension
AR: Artrite Reumatoide
CTD: Connective Tissue Disease

CHF: Cardiac Heart Failure
IHD: Ischaemic Heart Disease
CBVD: Cerebrovascular Disease
CVD: Cardiovascular Disease
COPD: Chronic Obstructuve Pulmonary Disease
CRF: Chronic Respiratory Failure
RR-MS: Relapsing-Remitting Multiple Sclerosis
P-MS: Progressive Multiple Sclerosis

Fig. 18.2 Region of Lomardy's risk stratification Polygon of chronicity

Conclusions

The process employed in the Region of Lombardy in recent years has revealed a focus on acceptance of chronically ill patients and an awareness that the introduction of new technologies requires innovative, flexible models of care and organisation to respond to the evolution of medicine and of the population in general. Technology is not a goal in itself, and it is not technology that offers solutions to problems in healthcare and organisation. It is knowledge and management of prevention, diagnosis, care and rehabilitation that ought to drive the choice of the most appropriate and sustainable technology, both on the micro scale (the patient, the MMG healthcare provider) and on the macro scale of the entire healthcare system.

The new regional act confirms that "the various forms of integration currently available should be applied systematically and allowed to evolve on the basis of a consistent overall plan, implementing a proactive, integrated, multi-dimensional approach to the care of chronically ill patients". The spread of the CREG services into new areas, the adoption of tools for telemedicine, the integration with NRS and the introduction of local hospital units are all prodromes that need to be included in a network with an overall vision to permit optimal management of patients, based on different stages of the illness. In this framework, telemedicine plays an important role. We must therefore recall the document

"Telemedicina – Linee di indirizzo nazionali"[14] ("Telemedicine: National Guidelines") in which the regions are asked to define a "document for the supply of clinical care integrated with Telemedicine" and a "document for definition of the standards of service of the Telemedicine services provided, also taking into account the standards set at the national level". In this vision, telemedicine must become an organic part of the system, be sustainable and appropriate and be customised according to the type of patient and the pathology or pathologies.

Redesigning the regional healthcare system reveals the truth of what we said initially, that is, that the characteristics of today's world and the complexity, uncertainty and ambiguity of the system require solutions based on keywords such as frugality, speed and agility, which are difficult to implement in an industrial context and even more so in the context of public services. In healthcare, which requires an overall vision permitting clarity and sharing of solutions, as well as agility in responding to citizens and patients, the challenge is an even more difficult one. But we must face up to this challenge, because the changing world demands it and because, due to both the spread of technology and the changes underway in society, patients are becoming more and more "impatient" and less liable to tolerate inefficiency and unfairness.

Suggested Reading

1. Giordano A et al (2013) Home-Based Telesurveillance Program in Chronic Heart Failure: Effects on Clinical Status and Implications for 1-Year Prognosis. Telemed E-Health 19(8):605–612
2. Passmore B, O'Shea T, and Horney N (2010) Leadership agility: a business imperative for a VUCA world. People Strategy 33(4). Kail, Leading in a VUCA Environment, HBR Blog Network, November 3, 2010 through January 6, 2011
3. Vitacca M et al (2016) Home-based telemanagement in advanced COPD: who uses it most? Real-life study in Lombardy. COPD J Chron Obstruct Pulmon Dis 13(4):491–498. http://dx.doi.org/10.3109/15412555.2015.1113243
4. Regione Lombardia – Regional Act no. 23, August 11, 2015
5. Regione Lombardia, Libro Bianco sullo sviluppo del Sistema sociosanitario in Lombardia. Un impegno comune per la Salute, Milano 30 giugno 2014
6. "Telemedicine – National guidelines"– State/Regional Agreement of 20 February 2014

---

[14] "Telemedicine – National guidelines"- State/Regional Agreement of February 20, 2014.

Printed in the United States
By Bookmasters